Patient Safety and Managing Risk in Nursing

Transforming Nursing Practice series

Transforming Nursing Practice is the first series of books designed to help students meet the requirements of the NMC Standards and Essential Skills Clusters for degree programmes. Each book addresses a core topic, and together they cover the generic knowledge required for all fields of practice.

Core knowledge titles:
Series editor: Professor Shirley Bach, Head of the School of Nursing and Midwifery at the University of Brighton

Personal and professional learning skills titles:
Series editors: Dr Mooi Standing, Independent Academic Consultant (UK and International) & Accredited NMC Reviewer and Professor Shirley Bach, Head of the School of Nursing and Midwifery at the University of Brighton

Mental health nursing titles:
Series editors: Sandra Walker, Senior Teaching Fellow in Mental Health in the Faculty of Health Sciences, University of Southampton and Professor Shirley Bach, Head of the School of Nursing and Midwifery at the University of Brighton

You can find more information on each of these titles and our other learning resources at www.sagepub.co.uk. Many of these titles are also available in various e-book formats; please visit our website for more information.

Patient Safety and Managing Risk in Nursing

Melanie Fisher and Margaret Scott

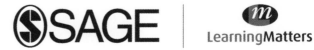
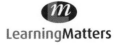

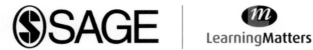

Learning Matters
An imprint of SAGE Publications Ltd
1 Oliver's Yard
55 City Road
London EC1Y 1SP

SAGE Publications Inc.
2455 Teller Road
Thousand Oaks, California 91320

SAGE Publications India Pvt Ltd
B 1/I 1 Mohan Cooperative Industrial Area
Mathura Road
New Delhi 110 044

SAGE Publications Asia-Pacific Pte Ltd
3 Church Street
#10–04 Samsung Hub
Singapore 049483

Editor: Alex Clabburn
Development editor: Eleanor Rivers
Production controller: Chris Marke
Project management: Diana Chambers
Marketing manager: Tamara Navaratnam
Cover design: Wendy Scott
Typeset by: Kelly Winter
Printed by Henry Ling Limited at
The Dorset Press, Dorchester, DT1 1HD

Library of Congress Control Number: 2013947936

British Library Cataloguing in Publication data

A catalogue record for this book is available from the British Library

ISBN 978-1-4462-6687-8 (hbk)
ISBN 978-1-4462-6688-5 (pbk)

MIX
Paper from
responsible sources
FSC
www.fsc.org   FSC™ C013985

Contents

Foreword

An essential component of nursing care is to ensure that patients' health improves and is maintained and that optimum health is achieved. This concept of nurses' caring is being extended by the current debate about patients who are suffering harm in our healthcare institutions. The shocking disclosures of the reports from the Mid Staffordshire NHS Foundation Trust Public Inquiry into conditions in hospitals have shone a disturbing light on patient safety in our healthcare systems. Nurses can no longer only ensure that their patients achieve optimum health: they also have a responsibility to make sure that their patients suffer no harm.

This new text in the *Transforming Nursing Practice* series provides students and qualified staff with a concise account of the responsibilities and roles of healthcare professionals in ensuring patient safety. It is timely and highly relevant to contemporary nursing practice. The concept of patient safety is examined in the context of the patients' needs in the twenty-first century. This book provides an excellent guide to understanding how mistakes occur and how, as professionals, we can address them.

By taking a journey through the history of patient safety and risk management the reader will see how a transparent and proactive approach has been developed to minimise safety incidents. The text looks at evidence-based research and policy drivers in relation to managing risk and applies this to practice scenarios. Error prevention models and root cause analysis are discussed, and safety and medicines administration errors examined thoroughly through the lens of the professional codes of conduct and responsibility.

Melanie Fisher and Margaret Scott, with John Unsworth, introduce the reader to the concept of safeguarding and raising concerns. These are issues that have not always featured in nursing courses and do need to be addressed from a wider perspective and applied to all healthcare settings. The authors introduce the reader to the role that human factors play in 'error'. This includes exploring the relationship between technical and human error. Measuring safe care can be challenging. The methods that can be used effectively are discussed and this includes the role of patients' complaints. From an organisational point of view consideration is given to the role culture plays in relation to patient safety and how leadership, at all levels of the organisation, can shape and ensure a positive and common culture.

Patient safety is an emerging healthcare discipline that underlines the importance of reporting, analysing and preventing harm to patients. This text will provide readers with a comprehensive insight into this subject, and how individuals can play a part in preventing and reducing patient harm as an integral part of their nursing responsibilities.

Shirley Bach
Series Editor

About the authors

Melanie Fisher LLM (Medical Law), MA (Education and Practice), PGDE, BSc (Hons), RN, ONC is Senior Lecturer and Programme Leader, Pre-registration Health Studies, Faculty of Health and Life Sciences, Northumbria University, Newcastle upon Tyne.

Melanie has worked in Higher Education for 13 years. Prior to this she worked in Adult Nursing, predominantly in Trauma and Orthopaedics, before taking up leadership and management roles that incorporated managing risk, promoting patient safety and developing practice. She has a keen interest in medical and healthcare law and has also worked with strategic commissioners as a patient safety associate.

Margaret Scott LLM (Medical Law), PGDAPL, BSc, RN is Senior Lecturer and acting Programme Leader, Pre-registration Health Studies, Faculty of Health and Life Sciences, Northumbria University, Newcastle upon Tyne. She has recently been accepted as a Fellow of The Higher Education Academy.

Margaret has 29 years' nursing experience, having worked predominantly in operating departments and anaesthetics prior to moving into nurse education. She is very safety focused due to working for many years in such a high-risk work environment and is committed to raising awareness and making a difference in providing safer care.

John Unsworth PhD, LLM (Medical Law), MSc, BSc (Hons), BA, PGCE, RN, QN, NTF is Principal Lecturer, Pre-registration Health Studies, Faculty of Health and Life Sciences, Northumbria University, Newcastle upon Tyne.

John has 30 years' nursing experience, having worked predominantly in community nursing prior to moving into nurse education. He has a keen interest in patient safety and is committed to ensuring that students are both fit for purpose and fit to practise at the point of registration. John is a panel Chair of the Nursing and Midwifery Council Investigating Committee, which considers a range of allegations of professional misconduct and lack of competence and other health-related concerns. He is also a Trustee and Council Member of the Queen's Nursing Institute. In 2013 he was made a National Teaching Fellow for his work in simulation and related to student assessment.

Acknowledgements

The authors would like to thank the following people:

Martin Bromiley and his family for their kind permission to use the case study of the late Elaine Bromiley.

Staff and students of Northumbria University Faculty of Health and Life Sciences: module Developing Fields within Nursing.

Eleanor Rivers, development editor for Sage/Learning Matters.

Introduction

What is *Patient Safety and Managing Risk in Nursing* about, and who should read it?

This introduction provides information about who should read the book, what it is about, why it is important and how it is structured. A brief overview of learning activities and NMC standards is also given.

The purpose of this book is to introduce the reader to the concept of patient safety and managing risk in today's twenty-first century healthcare service. It is particularly timely as safety in our health service is never far from the attention of the media and public scrutiny. It is ideal for nursing students of all fields but is equally accessible for the new registrant and other healthcare professionals who wish to learn more about safety and risk. The book takes a look at how patient safety and risk management has developed over the years to where it sits today. We examine some of the factors that compromise patient safety and explore strategies to subsequently manage it.

Book structure

Chapter 1 introduces the reader to patient safety and explores what it means. We look at how patient safety was traditionally viewed in the last century to how it is received now. We provide an overview of issues in patient safety that will later be explored in subsequent chapters, such as the nature of error, policy drivers, reporting systems and the quality agenda. As throughout the rest of the book, there are a number of activities and case studies to help readers consider what safety means to them and relate this to their own practical experience in their clinical settings.

Chapter 2 discusses risk in healthcare and examines some of the strategies designed to assess and manage risk, for example checklists. We look at evidence-based research and policy drivers in relation to managing risk and apply this to practice scenarios. We consider ways of managing risk in our own practice by drawing on case studies and incidents where harm has occurred or could potentially occur.

Chapter 3 examines the kind of things that may go wrong and that lead to accidents and incidents. We discuss error prevention models and root cause analysis. In addition, we discuss the process of reporting incidents and mistakes, but we also acknowledge some of the barriers that may prevent healthcare professionals from admitting to errors.

Chapter 4 looks more specifically at safety and medicines administration errors. We discuss a wide range of causative factors and prevention in medicine errors. We focus on insulin administration as an example of transferable practices, which can promote safe administration of different types of medicines. We specifically look at the nurse's role in the safe administration of medicines and guide readers to policies and standards to promote their own safe practice.

Chapters 5 and 6 introduce readers to the concept of safeguarding and raising concerns. Patient safety is not solely about avoiding errors in care and treatment, it is also about promoting safety and recognising those who are vulnerable. Chapter 5 was included in the book because safeguarding is an important area in healthcare delivery and sits comfortably with risk management and raising concerns. Chapter 6 looks more specifically at raising concerns and professional regulation. The chapter defines the nature and scope of professional accountability and regulation as applied to nursing. It explains how professional regulators can hold practitioners to account and maintain professional standards.

Chapter 7 introduces readers to the role that human factors play in 'error'. We explore the relationship between technical and human error, and take a further look at the skills required to prevent errors. We look more closely at the nature of errors and we consider lessons taken from high-reliability organisations, such as aviation and the military, to help us avoid errors.

Chapter 8 considers the way in which we measure safe care and how this can be challenging. We will briefly consider how measuring mortality is used as an indication of the quality of care provided by hospitals. We explore how the number of complaints received by patients or carers, or the numbers of accidents and incidents that have occurred over a given period of time, are often used to measure how safe the care is that we deliver. Key aims of the Commissioning for Quality and Innovation (CQUIN) framework and the NHS Safety Thermometer tool will be explored, and the benefits for both practice and patients.

Chapter 9 looks at how personal values and beliefs can influence the ways in which we behave. We then move on to explore values and beliefs from a professional perspective and how cultures and subcultures emerge within large, complex organisations, such as the NHS. Consideration will be given to what role culture plays in relation to patient safety and how leadership, at all levels of the organisation, can shape and ensure a positive and common culture throughout. Your role as a leader of care and the leadership traits that you already demonstrate, but might not be aware of, will be identified and explored.

Chapter 10, the concluding chapter, is where we consider the way forward in patient safety and quality care. The report of the Mid Staffordshire NHS Foundation Trust Public Inquiry is discussed further with emphasis on some of its recommendations. We consolidate some of the skills required of healthcare professionals in order to prevent errors occurring, and ask readers to reflect on their own responsibilities and learning needs in order to develop as safe and professional practitioners.

Requirements for the NMC *Standards for Pre-registration Nursing Education* and Essential Skills Clusters

The Nursing and Midwifery Council (NMC) has established standards of competence that have to be met by applicants to different parts of the register. The standards are necessary for safe and effective practice. As well as these standards the NMC has also identified specific skills students must acquire at various points of their educational programme. These skills are known as Essential Skills Clusters (ESCs). This book is structured in a way that will help you understand and meet some of these competencies required for entry to the NMC register. The boxes refer to the latest NMC Standards, taken from *Standards for Pre-registration Nursing Education* (NMC, 2010a).

Learning features

Learning about topics such as safety and risk is not always straightforward and is often dependent on your personal experience and stage in your learning or career. In order to help you contextualise and connect with the subject matter, there are a number of features in this book designed to help you to participate in your own learning. The chapters contain activities, case studies, scenarios and exercises to help you reflect, think critically and develop your own learning style. Each chapter has suggested further reading and websites to help you explore the topic further. There is also a glossary of terms at the end of the book that provides an interpretation of terminology (in **bold**) with which you may be unfamiliar. The activities are designed to allow you 'time out' from reading so that you can reflect on your own knowledge and practice experience. You may do this either by engaging in further reading and searching or discussing with a peer. Some of the activities provide an outline answer at the end of the chapter but others require you to reflect personally. You may wish to use some of these activities as part of your personal development plan (PDP). You could write them up for your PDP or personal portfolio as part of your studies and use them later to reflect upon. Some of the further reading has been highlighted as beneficial for those of you preparing for interview.

The book is designed to be read from cover to cover or to 'dip in' and 'dip out' of. It is an introductory text but is useful as a springboard to further reading and understanding.

Chapter 1
Patient safety and quality

Chapter aims

After reading this chapter you will be able to:

- define what is meant by the terms 'patient safety', 'harm' and 'error';
- begin to understand how patient safety has developed in the UK and beyond;
- identify some of the key organisations involved in promoting and monitoring patient safety;
- demonstrate an understanding of the role nurses play in promoting the safety of others.

Introduction

It may seem a strange principle to enunciate as the very first requirement in a hospital that it should do the sick no harm.
(Florence Nightingale, 1860/1969)

Over 300,000 incidents in healthcare within the UK were reported to the National Reporting and Learning Service between October 2003 and June 2011.
(NPSA, 2011c)

This chapter aims to introduce you to the concept of **patient safety** in healthcare provision in the twenty-first century. In order to understand how mistakes can and do occur and subsequently how we can address them, it is beneficial for you to have some understanding of the terminology used when discussing patient safety, and the nature of incidents that occur and compromise patient safety. The chapter is also designed to encourage you to consider your roles and responsibilities in preventing harm and managing risk. We can see from the above quote from Florence Nightingale that the importance of safety was acknowledged in the early days of healthcare provision. However, it will become apparent that patient safety management has not always been accomplished in the last two centuries and until more recent times was conveniently disregarded when things went wrong.

It will be useful to glean some knowledge and understanding of the history of patient safety, which has led to the more transparent and proactive approach to minimising safety incidents today. This will help you to understand where safety sits in modern healthcare practice. We will examine why patient safety is high on the agenda in healthcare and explore some of the policy drivers underpinning safety initiatives, focusing upon the UK but also touching upon some other parts of the world. We will also provide some case studies to enable you to identify patient safety issues that may arise in your own practice and allow you to reflect on them. The World Health Organization (WHO, 2011) advises that students of healthcare need to understand how different systems impact on the quality and safety of healthcare. By systems we mean tools and processes to monitor and learn from safety incidents, and we will touch upon these in this chapter and throughout the book. The management of patient safety fits closely within the framework of **clinical governance** and the quality agenda and we will briefly explore this relationship.

Patient safety is not a stand-alone discipline but rather one that is integrated into all aspects of healthcare. It is the responsibility of all who come into contact with the individual in a healthcare setting, from the porter to the surgeon. It is a theme that runs through all nurse education courses (and other healthcare professional programmes) and it is embedded in mandatory training for staff at all levels. Because it is such an important concept, it is imperative that student nurses are introduced to the concept early and that it is at the foundation of everything you learn and practise. We are fortunate that we can learn from hindsight and ironically through the mistakes of others. Nursing undergraduates and graduates reading this book should dismiss any fears of making mistakes out of context, because to err is human. Instead they should embrace the wisdom to avoid the mistakes of others, and practise with confidence and evidence-based knowledge.

Hospitals do the sick no harm?

Patient safety is at the heart of quality care and the fact that care may fall short of this fills people with horror. Imagine if you or your loved one came to harm while undergoing treatment or care in hospital or in the community. In recent years there have been a number of reports of patients being harmed through medical or nursing **errors**, some of which are tragic and others at the very least **negligent**. Whether this is a reflection of worsening substandard practice or more robust reporting and data collection is a subject of debate and will be the subject of discussion in subsequent chapters.

> ### Case study
>
> *Norma is a 40-year-old school teacher with two school-age children. She has been awaiting a date for surgery to remove her gall bladder. When she finally does receive the letter inviting her for the procedure, although relieved that her problem will be treated, she also feels apprehensive. She is very worried about the procedure, which will require an anaesthetic. She has only ever been admitted to hospital for the birth of her two children and although this was uneventful she has a morbid fear of hospitals. She has heard stories from colleagues and the media about 'things going wrong' and she is terrified that this will happen to her.*

> ### Activity 1.1   *Reflection*
>
> - Make a list of the things Norma may be anxious about.
> - If you were to be admitted to hospital for an invasive procedure, is there anything that you would be afraid of? If yes, make a list.
>
> *An outline answer is provided at the end of the chapter.*

The case study above was designed to get you to think about safety from a patient perspective. Perhaps your list in response to Activity 1.1 may be influenced by stories and reports in the media, television documentaries, your own experience or experiences of those close to you. It could be influenced by your experience of working in healthcare and insider knowledge. Perhaps you are aware of statistics regarding **adverse incidents** made available by government bodies.

Patient safety is certainly an issue that is discussed in a more open and transparent way than it was some years ago. Incidents that affected patient safety more than two or three decades ago were often left unreported and at best dealt with 'in house' (Vincent, 2010). It was deemed not to be in the public interest to talk about 'such things' as the image of medicine would be tarnished and public trust would dwindle. Medicine and healthcare have inherently been concepts that carry a plethora of risks and nursing the sick is no exception. However, the concept of keeping patients safe during their trajectory of care is indeed the essence of care and for medical staff it is grounded in the Hippocratic Oath to 'do no harm'. With hindsight it seems obvious that care and cures were sometimes worse than the illnesses themselves but, if harm did occur, it was usually unintended or accidental. There are of course some exceptions to this, notably nurse Beverly Allitt and Dr Harold Shipman, who were both convicted of murdering patients in their care. In addition, as healthcare technologies, knowledge and techniques develop, one can ask whether risk increases too. Vincent (2010) reminds us that the terms 'harm' and 'error' are sometimes equated when discussed in literature, but errors do not all lead to harm and not all harm is caused by error. It is important to keep this in mind and think critically about issues that involve risk and safety.

Harm and medical iatrogenesis

A term you may have encountered is **medical iatrogenesis**. This term is used to refer to disease or harm introduced by the physician. Translated, iatrogenesis comes from *iatros*, the name for a Greek physician, and genesis, meaning origin (Illich, 2002). Illich was a priest and philosopher who wrote prolifically on the subject, terming it 'medical nemesis'. His writings described the disabling impact of medicine and treatment upon health. Illich's controversial views implied that, by medicalising illness and health, doctors in particular have moved beyond their proper boundaries and by doing so have potentially caused harm. It is for individuals to arrive at their own conclusions about Illich's views. There is no doubt that, for some, treatment can be worse than the disease or illness itself. But the individual has to decide whether the outcome is worth it. Illich's thoughts are interesting but have to be balanced against the great benefits medical advances have brought over the past few decades. We mentioned earlier that not all harm is caused by error. Some treatments and interventions, for example chemotherapy, may cure cancer but, in the process, compromise the patient's immune system and induce severe nausea and vomiting, which is distressing and potentially harmful to some.

Activity 1.2   *Reflection*

- Think about some of the side effects patients may experience during the course of their treatment that are not caused by error but rather are an expected occurrence and outcome of established interventions.

An outline answer is provided at the end of the chapter.

Errors

Errors that do incur harm of course do happen in the delivery of care and can be **human errors** (caused by an individual or individuals) or technical errors (caused by device malfunctions). There has undoubtedly been an improvement in the way incident information is reported, recorded and disseminated in more recent years, so we have a greater understanding of the nature and trends that underpin patient safety events. In the later part of the last century, patient safety featured 'implicitly' in healthcare. Since the beginning of this century, patient safety is now 'explicit' and is linked to the quality agenda (as we explore in later chapters). There are a number of reasons for this, which will be discussed throughout the book. What, then, do we mean by patient safety and do all errors inevitably lead to harm?

Case study

Ahmed, an experienced community mental health nurse, visited James, a 32-year-old man with a long history of bipolar disorder. He spent some time discussing how James was feeling and he chatted to him about his new medication, which appeared to be having a positive effect on his mood. James had experienced behavioural problems in the past and his low mood and depression could be triggered by events that may seem trivial to others, but are meaningful to him. Ahmed left James to visit his next client, satisfied that everything was well. As he drove out of the road, he realised that he had mistakenly left James's case notes in the kitchen. His spine froze as he imagined how James may react if he was to read some of the records. Hurriedly he returned to the house and James was surprised to see him. He apologised to James that he had left something in the kitchen. James was unperturbed and said 'oh, no problem mate'. Ahmed retrieved the notes and bid him farewell. It appeared James was unaware his notes had been left and therefore had probably not read them. Ahmed was shaken at the thought of what may have potentially happened in this situation and became extra vigilant about managing case notes.

This was an error of judgement that thankfully had no serious consequences. However, had James accessed his notes, he may have read entries that could have been sensitive and triggered an exacerbation of his depression and anxiety.

So far we have discussed patient safety as a concept without defining it. As with the terms harm and error, it is not always clear exactly what it means. What, then, do we mean by patient safety?

How do we define patient safety?

Patient safety is defined by Vincent as: *the avoidance, prevention and amelioration of adverse outcomes or injuries stemming from the process of healthcare* (2010, p31). There are many definitions in the literature but this is perhaps the most succinct. Interestingly, now that patient safety is recognised as a concept, it has developed its own terminology, which will be defined throughout the chapters and in the glossary.

Activity 1.3   *Evidence-based practice*

You listed your fears about what may potentially go wrong in healthcare in Activity 1.1.

- Now make a list or discuss with a fellow student, mentor or colleague the types of errors that *actually* occur and are reported.

An outline answer is provided at the end of the chapter. Further data and statistics will also be explored throughout the book.

Your discussion may have been based on your own experiences, observations or anecdotal evidence. You may have also given some thought to errors that compromised patient safety and those that did not result in harm.

The development of safety in the UK and beyond

Patient safety is a concept that is acknowledged and addressed globally. The United States has long been aware of patient safety as an issue, in the main due to **litigation** and the financial cost of mistakes. Other countries, including the UK, have been quick to follow and the media have probably had some part to play in this. In the UK, the media are influential and court public opinion. Mistakes in healthcare that reach the headlines sell papers and boost viewings. The public are interested in what 'goes on' in hospitals, care homes and in social care, even though a good proportion of reports tend to highlight shortcomings in care delivery. The public have greater expectations when it comes to healthcare as they have greater access to information about illness, treatment and services via the media and internet technology. However, because not all information available to us is credible, this can cause confusion and lead to individuals being misinformed.

Activity 1.4   *Critical thinking*

Some newspaper headlines print statements such as: 'Patients are starving in our hospitals!' and 'Woman left to die in a corridor.' Think about the potential effect on members of the public reading this.

- Do you think media reports are always factual?
- Do all journalists reporting these stories understand the context and complexities associated with healthcare delivery?

Outline answers are provided at the end of the chapter.

Raising awareness of patient safety

Culture in society and healthcare is changing; the days of 'doctor knows best' are diminishing.

While the notion of medical **hierarchy** is still evident in some communities, patients are much more likely to question health professionals and reject perceived substandard care. Perhaps the most influential catalyst to the development of patient safety was the publication of the US Institute of Medicine's 1999 report, *To Err is Human*. It raised political and public awareness in the United States. The Institute called for a national effort to address safety in healthcare and recommended that a centre for patient safety should be established within the Agency for Healthcare Research. This report and subsequent response from the Government spurred other governments to take action and, in 2000, Sir Liam Donaldson, the Chief Medical Officer for the Department of Health, led on the production of the UK's equivalent report: *An Organisation with a Memory* (OWAM; DH, 2000a).

In the UK, prior to the publication of OWAM, there had been some notable incidents that were starting to put patient safety into the spotlight. The Bristol Royal Infirmary 'scandal' was seen as a high-profile incident and catalyst for change in the way incidents are reported and managed.

Case study

Lack of openness and transparency masked the substandard practice of paediatric heart surgeons at the Bristol Royal Infirmary (BRI). In the late 1980s some clinical staff became concerned about the poor outcomes of children who underwent cardiac surgery, compared with the outcomes of other specialist units, and 'blew the whistle' (an unprecedented action for its time and one that will be discussed later in this book). An external enquiry was ordered and the case received a plethora of media attention. Some of the parents complained to the General Medical Council (GMC), which in 1997 examined the cases of 53 children, 29 of whom had died and 4 of whom had suffered brain damage. An enquiry was ordered and chaired by Professor Ian Kennedy and a report published in 2001 (BRI, 2001). Three doctors were found guilty of serious professional misconduct and two were struck off the register. The anaesthetist who blew the whistle left the UK for Australia.

Activity 1.5   *Critical thinking*

- Why do you think the substandard practice described in the BRI case study went on for so long before it was reported?
- Do you think the same situation would be reported earlier if it happened today?

One would hope that today an incident such as this would be intercepted earlier. The next few paragraphs outline why.

The role of the National Patient Safety Agency

Following the publication of OWAM, the Government responded to the need for safer care by setting up the arm's-length body, the National Patient Safety Agency (NPSA). The agency is responsible for leading and contributing to safe patient care by informing, supporting and influencing organisations and people working in the health sector. They have three divisions:

- National Reporting and Learning System (NRLS): concerned with identifying and reducing risks to patients receiving NHS care and leading on national initiatives to improve patient safety;
- National Clinical Assessment Service (NCAS): supports the resolution of concerns about the performance of individual clinical practitioners to help ensure their practice is safe and valued;
- National Research Ethics Service (NRES): protects the rights, safety, dignity and well-being of research participants who are part of clinical trials and other research in the NHS.

In 2010–11, the Government reviewed arm's-length bodies in an effort to drive
istration costs and reduce bureaucracy in the health service. It recognised the value
functions and recommended it should be abolished but with its functions continui
ways. The patient safety division will be incorporated into the new NHS Commiss

Patient safety incident data

The NRLS collects confidential reports of patient safety incidents across England and Wales
through a national reporting system. Common themes and risks are analysed by safety experts
and clinicians so that lessons can be learned and disseminated across healthcare organisations.
This can be through safety alerts, tools to promote a strong safety culture and national initiatives
in specific areas of high risk: *Through its funding and monitoring of the three independent National
Confidential Enquiries (patient outcome and death, maternal and child health, and suicide and homicide by people
with mental illness), the NRLS can maximise the benefits of their in-depth research to better improve care* (NPSA,
2008c, p19). An example of one initiative that developed as a result of such research was the
adult patient's passport to safer use of insulin. This safety alert is aimed at improving patient
safety by empowering patients to take an active role in their treatment with insulin through the
use of patient-held records that will be shared with healthcare professionals involved in their care.

You may be aware of other organisations that collect and record data relating to patient safety
incidents. It has to be said that reporting systems in healthcare can be confusing and daunting.
You may get lost in the swamp of organisations, bodies and departments that you read and hear
about. Vincent (2010) supports this view and suggests that, ironically, reporting systems lack
cohesion and integration and duplicate functions, and that many organisations support multiple
systems.

Other reporting systems

Reporting systems operate at different levels within the healthcare system. Some operate at local
level through the hospital/Trust risk management and clinical governance framework. Incidents
are reported locally using a standard incident form. Incidents that are reported are not always
errors, but urgent action can then be taken to prevent harm to patients. Incidents can be used as
triggers to allow for reflection and to improve and develop practice. Typical examples of incidents
that nurses may have been required to report include medicines administration errors, patient
falls and faulty medical devices. The information will be processed using organisation-specific
systems and subsequent action will be determined by the nature and consequences arising from
the incident. Other reporting systems operate at regional or national level and have different
audiences depending on their level of operation. For example, the Medicines and Healthcare
products Regulatory Agency (MHRA) is concerned with medical devices and medicine products
that have contributed to error. Professional regulatory bodies (Nursing and Midwifery Council
(NMC), General Medical Council (GMC) and Health and Care Professions Council (HCPC))
are interested in individuals on their registers who may be practising in a negligent manner.
Incident reporting systems are reliant upon individuals but, as we will see in subsequent chapters,
reporting systems are not a panacea for preventing harm.

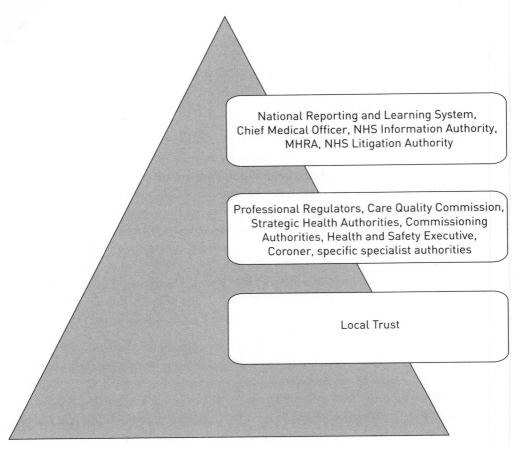

National Reporting and Learning System, Chief Medical Officer, NHS Information Authority, MHRA, NHS Litigation Authority

Professional Regulators, Care Quality Commission, Strategic Health Authorities, Commissioning Authorities, Health and Safety Executive, Coroner, specific specialist authorities

Local Trust

Figure 1.1: Examples of British authorities who may receive reports (these organisations change from time to time with NHS reforms)

In Scotland, patient safety is guided by Healthcare Improvement Scotland, a health body formed in April 2011 and concerned with quality and excellence in healthcare delivery. In Ireland at the time of writing, they too have their own national patient safety agenda (see www.patientsafety first.ie). Find out what systems your own healthcare placement provider feeds into. Figure 1.1 provides examples of authorities requiring safety incident information, but is by no means a complete list.

There are, of course, a number of strategies and tools to assist with the monitoring of data and management of safety incidents. We will explore these in later chapters.

Clinical governance and the quality agenda

So far we have discussed the development of patient safety in the UK in relation to reporting patient safety incidents. Another key development in patient safety is the growth of clinical governance and the quality agenda (DH, 2010a). You may be familiar with the terms 'clinical governance' and 'quality', but you may not be fully conversant with what they mean in relation to healthcare. The concept of clinical governance is linked to New Labour's first White Paper on health: *The New NHS: Modern, dependable* (DH, 1997). The aim of the paper was to reform the health service by improving quality and discarding failed policies that had prevented it working effectively in the past. This was prompted by a number of factors, including demographical changes in the population, increases in complaints going to litigation, changes in care and advances in technology. Clinical governance in healthcare is a term used to bring the whole quality agenda together in healthcare organisations. Much has been written on the core principles of clinical governance, but essentially the key components as defined by McSherry and Pearce (2002) are:

* ensuring quality improvement and maintenance;
* fostering a culture (organisational philosophies, belief and behaviours);
* ensuring safety;
* maintaining professional and organisational accountability.

All healthcare Trusts have a framework of governance embedded in the organisation, and within the framework is a component of risk management that is concerned with practising safely, and reducing clinical and non-clinical risks (we will explore risk management further in Chapter 2). It is obvious, therefore, that reducing and eliminating patient safety incidents will contribute to the quality of care. Governance also recognises the responsibility and accountability required of the organisation in the planning and delivery of care.

Activity 1.6   *Research and evidence-based practice*

* Find out about the clinical governance framework in your own Trust.
* Do you think it impacts on your own role? If so, then how?

As this activity is based on your own observations, there is no answer at the end of the chapter.

What is quality?

We use the term 'quality' frequently in everyday life and there are a number of lay definitions. For example, quality is defined as *degree of excellence* by the *Oxford English Dictionary* (2010) and *how good or bad something is* by the *Cambridge Dictionary* (2010). Quality has long been an important criterion in the purchase of retail products. More recently, however, it is also associated with public and private service providers in competitive and publicly scrutinised organisations, where the public have increasingly high expectations of the type of quality or service they can expect. Undoubtedly access to the internet has increased the availability of information and therefore expectations. Alongside this there are many social networking sites and blog sites where personal opinion is shared in the public domain.

Quality in healthcare has its own meaning, which it is important for you to understand. Donabedian (2003) has written extensively on quality in healthcare and suggested that it is dependent on technical excellence and the manner and humanity in which care is delivered – all of these are core attributes in nursing. The White Paper, *The New NHS: Modern, dependable* (DH, 1997), suggested that a quality organisation can be achieved by proactively ensuring that the following processes and attributes are present.

- An integrated approach to quality assurance is present throughout the whole organisation.
- Leadership skills are developed in line with clinical professional needs.
- Infrastructures that foster the development of evidence-based practice are present.
- Innovations are valued and good practices are shared within and outside the organisation.
- Clinical risk management systems are in place.
- A proactive approach exists in relation to reporting and learning from **untoward incidents**.
- Complaints are taken seriously and actions are taken to prevent recurrence.
- Poor clinical performance needs to be recognised in order to prevent harm to patients.
- Practical and professional development are aligned and integral to clinical governance frameworks.
- Clinical data are of the best quality and can be used effectively to monitor patient care and clinical outcomes.

Reflect on your own organisation where care is delivered to see if you can identify how these principles are integrated into the organisational culture. Think about how your own role as a nurse might contribute to these aspects of a quality organisation. The next section of this chapter will begin to explore your role in patient safety, but this is returned to throughout the book.

Your role as a nurse in promoting the safety of others

Case study

David is a second-year student nurse on placement in an elderly care ward in a hospital for people with learning disabilities. There has been an outbreak of clostridium difficile, resulting in some patients being nursed in isolation cubicles and others put together in a four-bed bay. There is an infection control policy in place, but David has observed something that disturbs him. He has noticed that the ward manager constantly wears a wristwatch. He is aware that this is in breach of uniform policy and also presents a risk of spreading infection. He is unsure how to address this situation and ponders over the choices of action available to him.

If you are a student nurse in a clinical environment, you are a junior member of staff but an important member of the team. Dealing with situations such as the one above can make you feel uncomfortable, but you also have a duty of care to patients and those whom your actions or omissions may affect. Policies and procedures are there for a reason. You, the student, as well as registered nurses are bound by a contract of employment. Students have to adhere to the rules and regulations set out by the education provider and placement provider. You also must adhere to the codes set out by the NMC. You have a duty to *safeguard* patients. (We will discuss more about safeguarding in Chapter 5.)

Activity 1.7   *Critical thinking*

- What would be the most appropriate course of action for David to take?
- Do you think the response of the ward manager matters? Discuss with peers and supervisors.
- With consideration of the type of situation David has found himself in, what is your responsibility as a nursing student in relation to promoting patient safety?

Outline answers are provided at the end of the chapter.

How will you be involved in patient safety?

As a student nurse you are responsible for your actions. As a registrant you are accountable for your own actions and the actions of some others if you have delegated a task or activity to another individual. As a student nurse, you must maintain and promote patient safety from the very first day of commencing your course in accordance with the NMC *Standards for Pre-registration Nursing Education* and Essential Skill Clusters. Most pre-registration curricula will have explicit practice learning outcomes developed around patient safety. You will also be provided with information and evidence through the theoretical component of your educational programme. While your mentor and other registrants are accountable for what they ask you to do, you must also be aware of your own competence and limitations so that you avoid harming someone. You must also be aware of policies, procedures and guidelines. This can feel like wading through a swamp at first, but with experience and support you will become more familiar with expectations placed upon you. Figure 1.2 illustrates the arms of responsibility bestowed upon the student nurse.

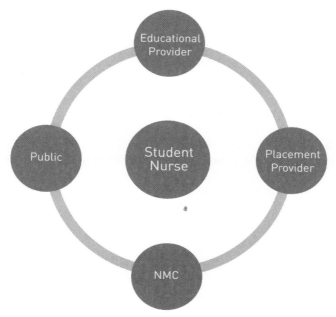

Figure 1.2: The responsibilities of the student nurse

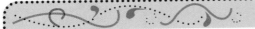

Chapter summary

This chapter has briefly introduced you to the concepts of patient safety quality. We have only touched the surface but you should now have an understanding of what is meant by patient safety and have gleaned some idea of the types of things that can go wrong when patients receive healthcare. You should now understand how and why safety has developed as a key focus within healthcare, and the main organisations involved in monitoring patient safety in the UK. You should also be giving thought to how you, as a professional practitioner, can help to reduce the risk of patient safety incidents and improve quality of care. The following chapters will explore some of the concepts mentioned in much more detail and, throughout the book, you will be provided with further reading and useful websites to enhance your understanding of this subject.

Activities: brief outline answers

Activity 1.1: Reflection (page 6)

You may have included the following in your lists:

- fear of anaesthetic;
- acquiring an infection;
- receiving the wrong medication;
- wrong site procedure;
- being a patient and feeling vulnerable;
- having to undress;
- lack of privacy;
- not being in control;
- fear of pain;
- fear of altered body image.

Activity 1.2: Reflection (page 7)

- After antibiotic therapy patients may experience nausea, skin irritation and other recognised side effects.
- Enforced bed rest increases the risk of pressure ulcers, muscle wasting and urinary infection.
- Side effects of some analgesics include diarrhoea and constipation.
- Chemotherapy can lead to hair loss in some patients.
- Radiotherapy can damage healthy tissue as well as diseased tissue.

Activity 1.3: Evidence-based practice (page 8)

According to the National Reporting and Learning System of the NPSA, the following incidents by type were recorded between April 2010 and March 2011 in England and Wales:

- medication;
- treatment, procedure;
- access, admission, transfer, discharge;
- documentation errors;
- infrastructure including staffing, facilities, environment;
- clinical assessment and diagnosis;

- disruptive behaviour;
- consent, communication, confidentiality;
- self-harm behaviour;
- medical devices;
- infection control;
- patient abuse by staff/third party.

Activity 1.4: Critical thinking (page 9)

Stories about healthcare interest the public and sell newspapers. While some media coverage of events can be factual and accurate, some accounts fall below this standard. Although you as a student or registrant may read articles and analyse them using your own judgement, the lay person may not have this ability and forms an opinion based on what he or she has read.

Activity 1.5: Critical thinking (page 10)

Whistleblowing is recognised as essential, if patient safety is likely to be compromised by substandard practice. However, the acceptance of whistleblowing is a relatively new concept, acknowledged by organisations and professionals. At the time of the inquiry, it was considered to be 'not the done thing' to raise concerns about a professional's standard of practice. The concept is still viewed by some to be contentious and this is explored in later chapters.

Activity 1.7: Critical thinking (page 15)

You are required by the NMC to act in accordance with its codes of practice and this includes:

- acting professionally and in accordance with policies and procedures;
- being knowledgeable and recognising your limitations;
- reporting incidents and occurrences in accordance with policy;
- acting without delay if you suspect patient safety is compromised.

The ward manager is an important figurehead in the clinical domain and, as well as the duties imposed on him or her by the professional regulator, there is also an obligation to lead and deliver best practice. Some of you may feel comfortable in approaching the ward manager to discuss directly your concerns, although others may think it more appropriate to discuss them with their mentor.

Further reading

Griffith, R and Tengnah, C (2010) *Law and Professional Issues in Nursing*, 2nd edition. Exeter: Learning Matters.

An accessible, easy-to-read book to help you understand your obligations in law as a nurse. Chapter 13 on health and safety is particularly helpful if read alongside this chapter.

McSherry, R and Pearce, P (2002) *Clinical Governance: A guide to implementation for healthcare professionals.* Oxford: Blackwell Science.

Chapter 2 provides an overview of clinical governance, explaining what it is and how it has been implemented in the NHS.

Northway, R and Jenkins, R (2013) *Safeguarding Adults in Nursing Practice*. London: Sage/Learning Matters.

This book will help you understand the concept of safeguarding, which links explicitly to patient safety.

Vincent, C (2010) *Patient Safety*, 2nd edition. Chichester: Wiley Blackwell.

Chapter 5 discusses reporting and learning systems and offers the reader further detailed information on this subject.

Useful websites

www.doh.co.uk

The Department of Health website is a general, useful resource as it provides news and information on the latest developments in patient safety. You can access archived as well as current reports such as OWAM.

www.npsa.nhs.uk

Th NPSA website provides an overview of the organisation's function. It also provides data on incident reporting.

Chapter 2
Risk and healthcare

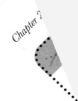

NMC Standards for Pre-registration Nursing Education

This chapter will address the following competencies:

Domain 1: Professional values

1. All nurses must practise with confidence according to *The Code: Standards of conduct, performance and ethics for nurses and midwives* (NMC, 2008), and within other recognised ethical and legal frameworks. They must be able to recognise and address ethical challenges relating to people's choices and decision making about their care, and act within the law to help them and their families and carers find acceptable solutions.
4. All nurses must work in partnership with service users, carers, families, groups, communities and organisations. They must manage risk, and promote health and well-being while aiming to empower choices that promote self-care and safety.
7. All nurses must be responsible and accountable for keeping their knowledge and skills up to date through continuing professional development. They must aim to improve their performance and enhance the safety and quality of care through evaluation, supervision and appraisal.

Domain 2: Communication and interpersonal skills

2. All nurses must use a range of communication skills and technologies to support person-centred care and enhance quality and safety. They must ensure people receive all the information they need in a language and manner that allows them to make informed choices and share decision making. They must recognise when language interpretation or other communication support is needed and know how to obtain it.

Domain 4: Leadership, management and team working

6. All nurses must work independently as well as in teams. They must be able to take the lead in co-ordinating, delegating and supervising care safely, managing risk and remaining accountable for the care given.

This chapter will address the following ESCs:

Cluster: Organisational aspects of care

9. People can trust the newly registered graduate nurse to treat them as partners and work with them to make a holistic and systematic assessment of their needs; to develop a personalised plan that is based on mutual understanding and respect for their individual situation promoting health and well-being, minimising risk of harm and promoting their safety at all times.

10. People can trust the newly registered graduate nurse to deliver nursing interventions and evaluate their effectiveness against the agreed assessment and care plan.

12. People can trust the newly registered graduate nurse to respond to their feedback and a wide range of other sources to learn, develop and improve services.

14. People can trust the newly registered graduate nurse to be an autonomous and confident member of the multi-disciplinary or multi agency team and to inspire confidence in others.

17. People can trust the newly registered graduate nurse to work safely under pressure and maintain the safety of the service users at all times.

18. People can trust the newly registered graduate nurse to enhance the safety of service users and identify and actively manage risk and uncertainty in relation to people, the environment, self and others.

By entry to the register:

9. Reflects on and learns from safety incidents as an autonomous individual and as a team member and contributes to team learning.

11. Assesses and implements measures to manage, reduce or remove risk that could be detrimental to people, self and others.

12. Assesses, evaluates and interprets risk indicators and balances risks against benefits taking account of the level of risk people are prepared to take.

14. Works within policies to protect self and others in all care settings including the home care setting.

After reading this chapter, you will be able to:

- identify some areas of foreseen risk that you have observed in your clinical environment;
- begin to understand how to assess and manage risk within healthcare delivery;
- understand the relevance of policy/procedure that may influence your practice;
- consider the importance of reporting incidents within the clinical environment;
- comment on why managing risk is important in relation to patient safety;
- understand how agreed standards can reduce risk;
- begin to understand the value of checklists in healthcare delivery.

Introduction

Healthcare delivery is a risky business and, although we acknowledge that it is impossible to eradicate all risk, there are many activities and actions that can be introduced to reduce opportunities for error and the potential to cause harm and negative incidents. Through identifying and managing situations or actions that put patients at risk from harm, improvements can be made to the quality and safety of healthcare services, and ultimately patient outcome. The purpose of this chapter is to enable you to explore, within your own clinical environment, some of the issues that can contribute to errors being made, or to harm occurring. Strategies to manage and avoid healthcare risk and errors will be examined, including the value of a standard evidence-based approach to ensure that treatment, care or the process is safe and effective, with a positive outcome for the patient. Recognising the opportunity to act proactively to avoid problems, as opposed to reacting to problems as they appear, is a key skill in the identification and management of risk. Perhaps the most important skill nurses can have, however, is the ability to understand and manage themselves in such situations.

Foreseeable risk

In simple terms foreseeable risk is a term used to anticipate the likelihood of injury or damage associated with a given set of circumstances. For example, a skier hits a bump on a ski run, falls and badly breaks a leg. This is a foreseeable risk of skiing. Foreseeable risk is also an established legal term and forms part of the criteria that can be used to determine whether **negligence** or harm has occurred. Nurses have a legal duty to avoid foreseeable harm to others (see Chapter 10 of *Law and Professional Issues in Nursing* (Griffith and Tengnah, 2010)).

Case study

Norma attends the pre-assessment clinic prior to admission for gall bladder surgery. Not only does Norma undergo a physical assessment, but she also has the opportunity to discuss some of her concerns in relation to her forthcoming surgery. The Nurse Practitioner is able to explain the benefits of this particular surgical intervention but without hesitation also discusses the associated risks. At this point Norma feels a certain sense of relief as she is now able to make an informed decision. For Norma the benefits of the surgery far outweigh the risks.

Norma is admitted to the ward on the day of surgery. She has already signed her surgical consent form whereby the surgeon reiterated the associated risks. The anaesthetist assigned to her case has just started for the day and comes on to the ward to speak to Norma. He assesses Norma in relation to the anaesthetic and considers her to be 'low risk' with regard to any airway problems. He concludes that the anaesthetic to be delivered is routine and the potential for any harm to Norma is extremely low, although all anaesthetics carry an element of risk. Norma is content with this explanation. She has never had an anaesthetic before and doesn't really know what to expect.

Hospital protocol dictates that an anaesthetist at the beginning of each shift must check all anaesthetic equipment used in the operating theatre. Due to time pressures and the fact that the anaesthetist has three other patients to see and assess, the anaesthetist relies on the checks that the operating department practitioner has made and does not perform any additional checks himself.

Risk assessment and risk management

From this example we can identify some of the risks associated with healthcare delivery, but risk assessment and management of risk often involve the need to see the bigger picture – which may not always be evident to members of the team. In order to understand the challenges and benefits in relation to patient safety, it is necessary to understand something of the context of risk assessment and risk management. It is evident that terminology varies, but that the aims of clinical risk management and patient safety are the same: to reduce or eliminate harm to patients (Vincent, 2010). The following simple four-step process is commonly used to manage clinical risks.

1. Identify the risk.
2. Assess the frequency and severity of the risk.
3. Reduce or eliminate the risk.
4. Assess the costs saved by reducing the risk or the costs of not managing the risk.

Activity 2.1   *Critical thinking*

Take some time to consider the following questions.

- Before Norma can make an informed decision what does she need to consider?
- What areas of risk does Norma have little or no control over?
- Is there any potential for unnecessary risk that could be avoided?
- Do you think that there could be any potential to cause harm?
- What would you do if you knew that an individual had deviated from policy/protocol?

Outline answers are provided at the end of the chapter.

Managing risk plays a large part in healthcare and patient safety. Risk is the chance that any activity or action could happen and harm you. Almost everything that we do has associated risk, such as crossing the road or travelling by aeroplane. People will generally take risks if they feel that there is an advantage or benefit, so how does this apply to healthcare? When patients consider having a procedure, intervention or screening, they will need to know the benefits and risks or any uncertainties to help them make an informed decision. Should a patient decide to go ahead with a procedure, informed decision making will form the basis of his or her informed consent. To a large extent the patient has control of the situation, as he or she will have already given due consideration to the benefit of an action and whether or not that outweighs the risk. It is important to note that nurses and all healthcare professionals have a responsibility to warn patients of known risks, irrespective of size. If you fail to do so you may be liable to an accusation of negligence (see Chapter 10 of Griffiths and Tengnah, 2010).

Areas in which patients have little or no control over risk must also be considered, for example contracting methicillin-resistant *Staphylococcus aureus* bacteraemia during a hospital stay. It is not usually possible to eliminate all risks, but healthcare staff have a duty to protect patients as far as is 'reasonably practicable'. This means that you must avoid any unnecessary risk; however, we need to look at risks and benefits together. There is no such thing as a zero risk and it is best to focus on the risks that really matter – those with the potential to cause harm.

Research indicates that about 10 per cent, or approximately 900,000 patients a year, are harmed during healthcare encounters (Davis et al., 2008). An adverse incident may be defined as *an unintended injury or complication, resulting in prolonged hospital stay, disability at the time of discharge or death, caused by healthcare management/delivery, rather than the patient's underlying disease process* (de Vries et al., 2008). While most incidents do not result in permanent injury, they place a significant burden on patients and their families, who report poor experiences and adverse effects on their psychological and social well-being (NAO, 2004; NPSA, 2007d). In addition, the financial burden on the NHS is considerable, with an estimated healthcare spend of about £1 billion a year in the UK (WHO, 2004b).

Deviation from policies and protocols

In Activity 2.1 you were asked the following question.

- What would you do if you knew that an individual had deviated (sometimes referred to as a violation) from policy/protocol?

Your initial thought may be to report the incident. There are three types of incidents that should be reported:

- incidents that have occurred;
- incidents that have been prevented (also known as **near misses**);
- incidents that might happen.

Clearly deviation from hospital policy/protocol does not fit neatly into any of the above types of incident reporting. Deviating from policy/procedure in Norma's case may result in an incident, but the likelihood of an event resulting in harm would be low, therefore the need to report would probably not be considered prior to the administration of anaesthesia. The only time that such a deviation would feature in incident reporting systems is if there were serious consequences, which is very occasionally. Many deviations are in a sense invisible to those in the workplace, such as that identified within the case study. On a daily basis such deviations from protocol largely pass unnoticed and it is not uncommon for this type of deviation to go unreported; no one knows how often such deviations occur. Deviation is to some extent encouraged and tolerated in healthcare to deliver organisational efficiencies, but system flaws, poor understanding and insufficient peer control of reckless or overconfident individuals result in the boundaries of safe practice being breached on a regular basis (Amalberti et al., 2006).

There are many reasons why individuals deviate from following policy/protocol. Understanding why such negative behaviours pervade the NHS is explained in part because it is human nature sometimes not to follow rules, or to deviate from standard procedure, particularly in situations that are unusual and need to be managed. Other reasons for such deviations may include personal characteristics, such as laziness or poor time management. Organisational and cultural characteristics may contribute to deviation whereby complacency allows safety standards to be eased and finally ignored. Another consideration in relation to deviation from policy/protocol may be that there are competing demands in complex work situations; this type of deviation may not necessarily cause harm but relies very much on the intelligence and competency of the workforce delivering care; this could possibly be applied to Norma's case study.

The protocol highlighted in the case study defines a standard clinical procedure for a routine task. Protocols for routine tasks are standardised as variation is thought to be unnecessary and, on some occasions, dangerous. Protocols of this nature are equivalent to the safety rules of other industries whereby a required level of safety needs to be achieved. Such standard routines are the bedrock of a safe organisation (Vincent, 2010). Protocol-based care enables NHS staff to put evidence into practice by addressing the key questions of what should be done, when, where and by whom at a local level. It provides a framework for working collaboratively within multidisciplinary teams.

It is important that clinical policies and protocols are easily understood and are universally standard throughout an organisation or a professional body (such as the NMC through its *Code*, or the GMC). Agreed standards cannot be overemphasised in relation to risk reduction. Understanding why something is done in a particular way in a given situation allows us to contextualise actions in the clinical setting.

As many of the challenges in relation to compliance relate to cultural and organisational issues, it is vital that the development of value-based improvement is supported by the executive board and delivered through effective clinical leadership and management (see *Leadership, Management and Team Working in Nursing* (Bach and Ellis, 2011, especially pages 30, 48 and 49).

How agreed standards can reduce risk

Case study

The porter arrives on the ward to collect Norma and escort her to the operating theatre. Norma is ready and appropriately prepared for theatre. A theatre **checklist** *has been completed and her notes, consent form and X-rays are available. A ward nurse accompanies Norma to theatre alongside the porter. Norma begins to feel very anxious at the prospect of an anaesthetic and the ward nurse tries to allay some of her fears. The theatre nurse once again completes the theatre checklist with the ward nurse present. No areas for concern are identified and Norma is taken into the anaesthetic room. The theatre nurse encourages Norma to relax. The operating department practitioner and the anaesthetist appear. The anaesthetic is administered and Norma drifts off to sleep. Unbeknown to Norma a Surgical Safety Checklist had been carried out prior to the start of the operating list.*

As human error is inevitable and the changing environment of the NHS becomes increasingly complex, there are many systematic approaches in place to standardise the quality of care delivered. It is important to note that the human mind does have limitations, meaning that errors can occur from inexperience, poor training, faulty reasoning or decision making, poor memory and poor communication. We do need to accept that as humans we make mistakes, and once we accept this, we can improve patient safety. It would make sense that clinical tasks should be designed accordingly, for example by breaking tasks down into simplistic steps or by using a checklist approach. The safety checklist concept has been an integral part of many industries that face highly complex tasks, such as aviation, and have been successfully transferred to healthcare. Ultimately, regardless of the nature of the approach, the principle purpose of their implementation is commonly error/risk reduction or adherence to best practice.

Activity 2.2   *Reflection*

- Think about occasions where you have used a checklist.

One example that you may want to consider is the 'cockpit drill', the checks you should perform before driving a car or vehicle. The 'cockpit drill' is designed to enhance both safety and comfort.

Another example would be to use a 'shopping list' when you visit the supermarket. Consider how frustrated you feel when you visit the supermarket without a shopping list only to arrive home and realise you have forgotten the very item that you went to the supermarket for in the first place. Although forgetting a shopping list does not impact upon safety, it highlights the fact that, if we visit the supermarket without a list, we are more likely to have a memory lapse, emphasising the fact that the human mind does have limitations.

As the aim of this activity is for you to explore and reflect upon your use of checklists in everyday situations, there is no answer at the end of the chapter.

If we routinely approach specific tasks in practice with a 'shopping list' mentality, or in a systematic way, the likelihood is that the occurrence of a patient safety incident will be greatly reduced. For example, if ten people go to the supermarket with a shopping list and on that shopping list there is milk, the likelihood is that everyone will come home with milk. There might be a variation in the volume of milk, but at least all ten people will bring milk home. The standardisation of practice reduces variations in the treatment of patients and improves the quality of care. Such approaches to standardisation in healthcare are not only based on clinical information about the individual patient taking into account beliefs, desires, opinions and priorities, but are influenced by evidence-based thinking, decision making and judgement of risk. Society's local and national health economy, ethics and law also add a dimension to the context in which decisions are made about the care delivered.

- Consider *local* influences in relation to standardisation of the quality of care delivered and of risk reduction in your area of practice.
- Consider *national* influences in relation to standardisation of the quality of care delivered and risk reduction in your area of practice.
- Can you identify any *global* influences in relation to standardisation of the quality of care delivered and risk reduction?

Outline answers are provided at the end of the chapter.

We have considered some of the benefits of standardising our approach to delivering care. As just discussed, one way of approaching care in a more standard and uniform way is through the use of checklists.

The value of checklists in healthcare

As the case study develops you will note that the term 'checklist' has been introduced. A checklist differs from other cognitive aids or protocols/procedure in that it lies somewhere between the knot in a handkerchief or a scribble on the back of your hand, and a protocol, which, as discussed, typically entails a set of sequential steps that should be followed in a particular order leading to a predetermined outcome. Checklists can have several objectives, including memory recall, standardisation and regulation of processes or methodologies, providing a framework for evaluation or as diagnostic tools (Scriven, 2000), the main purpose being that certain mandatory items are not forgotten. Think back to the example of the shopping list in Activity 2.2. Well-designed checklists can standardise what, when, how and by whom care interventions are delivered and can reduce error in routine and emergency situations. Additionally, a checklist can provide a framework to ensure that there is a universal approach to clinical and procedural requirements.

The safety checklist concept or effect has been an integral part of many industries that face highly complex and potentially life-limiting tasks such as aviation and engineering. It has been recognised that this checklist approach has the same potential to save lives and prevent morbidity in medicine as it does in aviation, by ensuring that simple standards are applied for every patient, every time. One working example on a global scale is the implementation of a Surgical Safety Checklist, which has been shown to enhance patient outcome and reduce patient risk (WHO, 2009). The checklist consists of three phases: 'sign in' (before anaesthesia), 'time out' (before an incision is made) and 'sign out' (before the patient leaves the theatre). The World Health Organization (WHO) has developed this checklist to improve patient safety in the operating room and reduce post-operative morbidity and mortality regardless of the healthcare system or the economic setting. The aim of the WHO checklist is that a standard evidence-based approach to patient care in every operating theatre worldwide is adopted. Those who have chosen to adopt the Surgical Safety Checklist, perhaps with modification for their own needs, have reported promising results in relation to improvements in patient safety. Checklists can therefore be seen as powerful tools to standardise approaches and create independent checks for key processes. In 2012, WHO launched a collaborative field-testing exercise to learn and share experiences in relation to developing another checklist. The WHO Safe Childbirth Checklist is a 29-item checklist tool that reminds and helps staff to follow best practice that is evidence-based, aiming to improve maternal, foetal and neonatal health. Each item within the checklist is an action that needs to be taken and if missed can lead to complications or death. WHO is encouraging this global safety programme to help minimise the most common and avoidable risks endangering mothers and babies at the time of birth, with the goal of saving lives.

You may well have come across other systematic approaches to care delivery, such as care guidelines, **bundles**, triggers and **algorithms,** while in the practice environment.

Activity 2.4   *Reflection*

Think of the last time you used a checklist, bundle, trigger, guideline or algorithm in your own area of practice. Think about the situation, the context and your relationship with the patient.

*   Did you carry out this systematic/standardised approach to care delivery on your own, or was it necessary to adopt a team approach?
*   On reflection, are you able to confirm that a systematic/standardised approach has the potential to reduce the risk of harm or an adverse event?
*   If a standard approach was not adopted, are you able to identify the potential negative outcome for the patient?

One simple example, which you may want to consider, and which is universal to all areas of clinical practice, is hand washing.

As the aim of this activity is for you to explore and reflect on your own practice in relation to the use of standardised approaches, there is no answer at the end of the chapter.

Intentional rounding as a standardised approach to care delivery

One example of a standardised evidence-based approach to care delivery is in the realm of ward rounds. In January 2011 the British Prime Minister called for changes in the way nurses deliver care. The Care Quality Commission (CQC) revealed that problems had been found with providing good nutrition and dignified care, particularly in relation to elderly people: of 100 hospitals inspected, 49 gave rise to minor, moderate or major concerns relating directly to nutritional standards. Concern had been expressed about the need to ensure that essential aspects of nursing care are consistently delivered. One recommendation was for NHS hospitals to implement hourly nursing rounds, to check on patients and ensure that their fundamental care needs are met – an approach known as 'intentional rounding' in the United

States. Within the UK some organisations refer to this type of activity as 'comfort rounds' or 'care rounds'.

The origins of this evidence-based structured approach lie in the United States, where the Studer Group identified that comfort or care rounds had the potential to improve patient safety and satisfaction scores as well as creating a less stressful and more productive environment for nurses to work in. Over 400 international healthcare systems have applied this approach and scripted protocols, which include competency checklists, as a means of reviewing direct caring behaviours. Key aspects of patient care are categorised into 'Four Ps' during the nursing rounds process.

- **Positioning**: assessing the risk of pressure ulcers and ensuring that the patient is comfortable.
- **Personal needs**: scheduling trips to the toilet to avoid risk of falls.
- **Pain**: asking the patient to describe his or her pain level on a scale of 0–10.
- **Placement**: making sure the items a patient needs are within easy reach, e.g. a drink.

Making hourly rounds can be viewed as a bundle of interventions that promote not only the comfort but also the safety of both patients and staff, akin to bundles for ventilator-associated pneumonia and catheter-related bloodstream infection (Halm, 2009). The shared knowledge of the content of a checklist allows those delivering care to support one another by cross-checking what is being done and in what order. Checklists may be implemented as a stand-alone intervention, but more often than not they are part of several other components that go together to improve the quality and safety of care.

Activity 2.5   *Evidence-based practice and research*

Consider comfort or care rounds as an approach to healthcare delivery.

- Within your own area of practice does this approach to caring exist either formally or informally?
- Explore the benefits and limitations of such an approach. Does one outweigh the other?
- What key points would you need to consider if you were to introduce such an approach within your own area of practice?
- What may the challenges for practice be?
- Would you need to include all patients or would this vary depending on the patient's clinical condition or level of care required?

Outline answers and thoughts are provided at the end of the chapter.

We have considered how using standardised evidence-based approaches to care delivery can offer consistency to our patients. Approaching care in this way is very much a systems approach, but we also need to consider how as individuals we can reduce human error.

Managing human error

There are two main ways to manage human error – first, as previously considered, the 'systems' approach, which includes:

- a standard approach to certain tasks in the form of a protocol, policy or **care bundle**;
- a checklists approach ensuring that mandatory items are not forgotten.

The second approach is that of the 'individual'. Certain tools and techniques can help individuals to formally evaluate the risks they may be faced with or the potential for harm to occur. One such tool is the 'three bucket' model, which will be described in the next section. The management of risk is most effective when a 'systems' and an 'individual' approach are combined. In order to understand each approach it is necessary to develop the essential skills to identify 'risky' situations.

Foresight training – the individual approach

Foresight training is a concept that aims to help nurses develop and practise the skills needed to identify situations where the safety of a patient may be compromised and an incident is more likely to occur. Foresight is having the ability to identify, respond to and recover from the initial indications that an incident involving patient safety could take place, and having this particular skill is relevant to nurses working in a variety of clinical areas such as primary care, acute care and mental health settings. The underlying principles of foresight training can be applied in many settings, with the emphasis on preventing an incident involving the patient rather than analysing why incidents have happened. In more simplistic terms foresight training could be described as having the required skills necessary to acknowledge the fact that the incident did not reach the patient and consequently no harm was caused.

A simple practical example would be that, during the course of the day, the order in which patients were to go to the operating theatre had been altered due to an unplanned emergency that required immediate surgical attention. You notice that the wrong patient is about to be sent to the operating theatre and promptly communicate this to the nurse in charge, therefore potentially preventing an incident that could have compromised patient safety.

Foresight training has been developed to:

- improve awareness of the factors that might cause harm to a patient;
- empower staff to intervene to prevent patients from suffering accidental harm;
- increase local learning by sharing experiences;
- improve understanding of 'risk-prone' and 'near-miss' situations, and what should be reported;
- help nurses and midwives to adopt a more proactive approach to managing complex, dynamic healthcare systems.

Foresight is the ability to:

- recognise potential risks to patient safety in the healthcare system;
- identify, and respond to, initial indications that a patient safety incident could take place;
- intervene, and recover, to prevent a patient safety incident.

Evaluating your situation and preventing harm – 'three bucket' theory

The 'three bucket' theory is a conceptual model for understanding and assessing potential risk to patient safety. In this model there are three areas, or 'buckets', that influence the likelihood of harm occurring. The three buckets are self, context and task (see Figure 2.1).

The more the buckets fill up, the greater the likelihood of an error or harm occurring. The amount of supposed risk or harm in each 'bucket' is rated in turn by the person evaluating the risk or potential to cause harm as (1) low, (2) medium or (3) high. Being aware of this is foresight, and using foresight gives you a chance to prevent an error before harm occurs.

Full buckets, or high scores, do not always lead to error, just as nearly empty buckets are no guarantee of safety. The buckets will never be completely empty as healthcare delivery always carries an element of risk – only the level of risk changes. The amount of content in all of the buckets provides an *estimation of the probability* of error or harm occurring. As the probability of error increases, this is when we need to acknowledge the risk by becoming more cautious and considering additional support or assistance. It is worth considering that each bucket may contain positive as well as negative factors. For example, you may have returned from a two-week holiday, you feel well rested and the environment where you work is familiar; the staff are all very supportive, but you are faced with a very complex task.

Use the 'three bucket' approach to evaluate the factors that might cause harm to a patient. Ask yourself the following questions.

- **Self** – how safely are you able to work? This bucket is of concern to the individual. For example, is he or she tired and does he or she have the necessary experience, competence and knowledge to deal with the demands at that time?
- **Context** – how safe is your working environment? This bucket represents all background factors, including the environment (noise distractions, interruptions, handovers), equipment failures, inadequate staffing, resources and time.
- **Task** – how error prone is the task you are carrying out? This bucket considers all factors related to the task at hand and includes the difficulty of the task, duration and the physical demands.

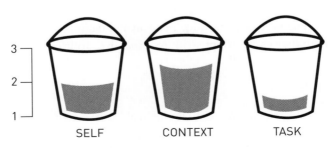

Figure 2.1: Diagrammatic representation of the 'three bucket' theory (adapted from NPSA, 2008d)

Consider the following questions in relation to self, context and task (adapted from James Reason's 'three bucket' model (NPSA, 2008d)).

SELF – how safely are you able to work?

Assess	Your level of knowledge, skill, experience and expertise.
	Your current capacity to do the task (fatigue, life events, illness).

- Are you working beyond your competence or training?
- Are you familiar with all staff, working practices, policies and protocols?
- Is this a job that you do so often that you do not have to think about it?
- Are you comfortable asking a question if you need to?

Ask yourself the following questions.

- Can you challenge senior staff?
- Have you had your break?
- Are you stressed or ill, or under the influence of alcohol or drugs?
- Are things outside work okay?
- How is your relationship with your line manager?

CONTEXT – how safe is your working environment?

Assess	Your physical environment and workspace, and the equipment to be used.
	Your team, management and organisation, and support network.

- How well do you know your working environment, and the equipment to be used?
- Is there enough space and light? Is the temperature okay? Is it noisy?
- Can you find and reach everything you need? Has the equipment been serviced?
- Are you trained to use the equipment you need, and is it easy to use?

Ask yourself the following questions.

- Do you have enough space to complete your task without being interrupted?
- Do you have enough time?
- How well do you know the people you are working with? Do you feel listened to and supported?
- Do you have enough information about what you are doing? Do you know what others are doing? Do they know what you are doing?
- Are you being pressured to do something you are not comfortable with?

TASK – how error prone is the task you are carrying out?

Assess	The complexity and novelty of the task, and the potential errors that could occur.
	The processes and procedures you need to follow.

- Is this a new task? Have you time to prepare?
- Do you feel confident to carry out this task?
- Have you ever made a mistake with this task before?
- Could you forget to finish this task, or forget where you are and have to start again?

- How likely is it that you would do steps to this task in the wrong order?
- Do you do this task so regularly that you might not notice if it goes wrong?

Ask yourself the following questions.

- How likely are you to notice if something unexpected occurs with this task?
- Do you know processes for rare, but possible events, such as power failure?
- Have new ways of working been introduced? What new risks are there?
- Are you likely to be distracted from your task? Can you plan to avoid this?
- Can you stop when you realise that you are juggling too many things at once?
- Is there a high risk, for example intravenous medication administration?

The case study below will provide an opportunity to explore how the 'three bucket' approach and foresight can be applied to the practice environment.

Case study

John Smith, a district nurse, has been a registrant for six months and has recently completed his preceptorship. Although Nurse Smith has worked weekends before, this is the first weekend that he has not had direct supervision from his preceptor. Nurse Smith is excited and looking forward to the challenge; he feels that his workload is manageable and that he has developed a good rapport with his patients. Before starting his home visits Nurse Smith calls into his base health centre to see if any messages have been left for him. When he arrives he is told that Sandra Peters, another district nurse, has called in sick and that he would need to see three of her patients. Nurse Smith agrees to visit the additional patients as he feels that he is competent to provide the necessary care. He does feel a little anxious as he had put a lot of planning into his own routine visits and allocated time based on each individual patient's care requirements. Nurse Smith now needs to prioritise his visits again, taking into consideration the additional patients.

Nurse Smith decides to visit Edna Green first. She is an insulin-dependent diabetic and she is also blind. Nurse Smith is conscious of the fact that she will need her blood sugar checked and her insulin administered before she can have any breakfast. When Nurse Smith arrives at Edna Green's home she is very upset because she has scalded her hand on hot water from the kettle. Nurse Smith reassures Mrs Green and asks her to sit down so that he can examine her hand. Fortunately, Nurse Smith believes the scald to be superficial, and dresses Mrs Green's hand appropriately. Nurse Smith takes care to document the treatment and dressing that has been applied to Mrs Green's hand. Mrs Green expresses her gratitude and thanks Nurse Smith as he leaves. Nurse Smith hurries to the next patient and feels pressured, as he had spent so much time with Mrs Green. It is only when he is leaving the second visit that he remembers he has not checked Edna Green's blood glucose or administered her insulin. He will need to go back.

This case study provides the opportunity to think about the foresight factors leading up to the incident in terms of the 'three bucket' model. You may find drawing the three buckets helpful at this stage (see Figure 2.1).

Foresight factors

Self

Level of knowledge
- Nurse Smith did not know the additional patients.
- There was no previous relationship between Nurse Smith and the additional patients – he was unable to appropriately assess individual care needs.
- Nurse Smith felt competent to visit the additional patients but his level of knowledge about each additional patient was limited.

Current capacity to do task
- Nurse Smith was stressed about the additional workload.
- Nurse Smith may have felt unable to challenge a more senior member of the team who allocated him the additional patients. Remember, Nurse Smith has only recently qualified.

Context

Workspace and equipment
- The environment was familiar to Nurse Smith, however the unexpected event created a diversion from why he was there in the first place.

Team and support
- Support structures were missing for Nurse Smith as this was his first weekend working on his own without his preceptor.

Organisation and management
- The organisation/management did not have time to find an additional member of staff to cover sickness.
- No concessions were made to the workload, given that the three additional patients were unfamiliar to Nurse Smith.

Task

Omission errors
- An unpredictable event that Nurse Smith did not plan for required immediate attention and interrupted the task of checking blood glucose and administering insulin.

Task complexity
- Nurse Smith was interrupted by the unpredictable creating a distraction.
- Nurse Smith was expected to juggle too many things at once. The additional workload had created stress and pressure on time allocation.
- The fact that Mrs Green had scalded herself needed immediate attention. Nurse Smith may not have felt confident to assess and dress the scald but did it anyway. He may have felt that he did not have time for additional care provision due to competing demands.

Task prioritisation

- Lack of experience may have meant that Nurse Smith was unable to prioritise tasks/visits appropriately.

Reflecting on the case study provides some indication as to how aspects of self, context and task can contribute to an incident that may compromise patient safety, and how awareness of these 'foresight factors' could have made a difference.

Activity 2.6   *Critical thinking*

Think about your own level of practice, competence and responsibility in relation to the following skills or tasks:

- administering an intramuscular injection;
- leading a medication (drug) round;
- a cardiac arrest situation;
- a blood transfusion;
- an attempted suicide;
- urinary catheterisation;
- hand washing;
- a theatre checklist;
- administration of buccal midazolam for prolonged epileptic seizure;
- confirming the correct placement of a nasogastric tube;
- nasogastric tube feeding under restraint;
- de-escalation;
- a self-harm situation.

Apply the foresight model of the 'three bucket' approach to each of the above skills or tasks considering your own level of knowledge, competence and responsibility.

Ask yourself the following questions.

- **Self** – how safely are you able to work?
- **Context** – how safe is your working environment?
- **Task** – how error prone is the task that you are carrying out?

Draw the buckets if you find this helpful.

As the aim of this activity is for you to explore and reflect on your own practice in relation to knowledge, competence and responsibility, there are no answers at the end of the chapter.

Both a 'systems' and an 'individual' approach have now been considered in relation to reducing human error and minimising risk. A 'systems' approach accepts that, as humans, we make mistakes and errors are to be expected. Countermeasures are put in place to trap errors and may take the form of an evidence-based, standardised approach such as a protocol or checklist.

Activity 2.7   *Reflection*

You may want to consider how many of the skills or tasks identified in Activity 2.6 are policy or protocol driven.

- How do policies and protocols influence your practice?
- Do policies and protocols reduce the likelihood of harm?
- What are the foreseeable risks and are they easily identifiable?
- Are you able to evaluate the factors that might contribute to a patient safety incident?
- Are you able to approach practice differently in order to prevent a patient safety incident?
- Have you established *insight* into *foresight*?

As this activity is based on your own research and reflections, there are no answers at the end of the chapter.

We have already mentioned why some people stray or deviate from policies and protocols. Errors generally occur when the policy or protocol is not known or has been forgotten. An example of this would be the re-sheathing of a needle after use. Although policy dictates that no needle should be re-sheathed after use, occasionally people forget and re-sheath the needle. They may be lucky and suffer no harm; they may be unlucky and receive a needle stick injury, which inevitably requires treatment and reporting. Deviation from a policy or protocol is usually conscious and, in terms of safety, reflects risk-taking behaviour, such as the example of the anaesthetist within the first case study about Norma (page 6). The key to reducing deviations or non-compliance would be to persuade those individuals responsible for such behaviour as to the necessity of adherence. This may be easier said than done, although steps may be taken to maximise compliance. First, all existing policies and protocols should be reviewed with regard to their relevance; they should be correct, comprehensible and readily available to all. Second, any unnecessary, out-of-date policies or protocols should be either abandoned or reviewed. Review dates should feature on all policies. Naturally compliance must also be achievable, and therefore due consideration must be given to realism, a sound evidence base and application to the situation. It should be noted that too many policies and protocols within an organisation could be stifling in relation to initiative and clinical decision making when a novel situation arises. However, protocol-based care should strive to reduce unnecessary variations in treatments and outcomes. It is not possible to develop a policy or protocol for every clinical dilemma, nor would it be appropriate to do so.

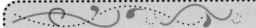

Chapter summary

In this chapter we have recognised that healthcare is inherently risky and, although it is impossible to get rid of all risk, there are many activities and actions that can be introduced to minimise opportunities for error or harm. Furthermore, this chapter has identified that no single approach to patient safety is sufficient to reduce all sources of harm associated with care delivery.

We have examined some of the contributing factors to incidents that may result in harm or disability. We have seen how the use of a standard evidence-based approach or process to routine tasks can minimise risk and provide the patient with a positive outcome.

This chapter provides a brief insight into how healthcare delivery can be a risky business and you are strongly recommended to access the useful websites or further reading to provide you with a more comprehensive understanding.

Activities: brief outline answers

Activity 2.1: Critical thinking (page 22)

*   Before Norma can make an informed decision, what does she need to consider?

Norma would need to consider whether the benefits of gall bladder surgery outweighed the risks. How you view risk depends to a large extent on your own circumstances and 'comfort zone'. How you view a risk is dependent upon one or more of the following.

*   The chance or frequency of the event occurring, for example post-operative haemorrhage or infection.
*   The chance of a condition being detected by a screening test (detection rate).
*   The benefits of the treatment or screening.
*   How much harm may be caused:
    *   if it is life threatening;
    *   if it is short term (temporary) or long term (permanent).
*   How much you feel in control of the decision.
*   How much you trust the person discussing the risk with you.
*   Whether you feel you understand the situation sufficiently.

Some of these factors will be more important than others. Concerns, anxieties and fears about the present and the future are very personal and may affect how risk is viewed. Risk can be given as numbers or words, or both. Some people may find it is more useful to discuss risk using pictures rather than words or numbers. It is very important that facts are discussed in a meaningful way. Good communication between yourself and the patient promotes a trusting relationship and assists the patient in taking more responsibility for decisions about his or her health.

*   What areas of risk does Norma have little or no control over?

Norma would have no control over contracting methicillin-resistant *Staphylococcus aureus* bacteraemia or *Clostridium difficile* infection, nor would she have control over an adverse drug event, for example, all of which are classified as major types of harm. Healthcare-associated infection (HCAI) is the commonest complication affecting hospitalised patients.

*   Is there any potential for unnecessary risk that could be avoided?

There is risk associated with the anaesthetist deviating from hospital protocol in relation to anaesthetic equipment checks.

- Do you think that there could be any potential to cause harm?

A malfunction of the ventilator or failure of any of the equipment that should have been checked by the anaesthetist could have potentially resulted in harm to Norma. Some other areas within the case study where there is potential to cause harm include:

- lack of diligence when checking Norma into theatre;
- non-adherence to equipment checks, e.g. diathermy equipment;
- anaphylactic reaction to antibiotic; staff uncertain of algorithm or drill to follow when an unexpected event occurs;
- haemorrhage during the operation resulting in Norma requiring an emergency blood transfusion.

This list is not exhaustive by any means but perhaps gives you some insight into the potential for something to go wrong. A lot of what we do can result in harm to patients; there is an element of uncertainty and we need to accept that a great deal of uncertainty will always remain. There is no doubt that patient safety is a risky business.

- What would you do if you knew that an individual had deviated from policy/protocol?

Your initial thought might be to report the individual to someone more senior, or your practice mentor.

Activity 2.3: Evidence-based practice and research (page 26)

A patient group directive (PGD) could be considered as a local influence that allows nurses and professionals allied to medicine to administer and supply medication directly to patients within a protocol.

National Service Frameworks (NSFs) may be considered as a national influence in relation to standardisation of care as they are policies set by the NHS. NSFs set clear quality requirements for care based on the best available evidence. The National Institute for Health and Care Excellence (NICE) is an independent organisation responsible for providing national guidance on promoting good health and preventing and treating ill health. In general, doctors, nurses and other healthcare professionals in the NHS are expected to follow NICE's clinical guidelines.

The World Health Organization (WHO) plays an essential role in the global governance of health and disease. Core global functions include establishing, monitoring and enforcing international standards.

Activity 2.5: Evidence-based practice and research (page 28)

Within your area of practice is care delivered in a consistent manner to reduce variation in clinical care and adverse incidents, for example two-hourly turning of bedfast patients, two hourly toileting, or support with feeding? If so, is this approach formalised by the use of documentation or do these activities occur as part of the everyday routine, thereby becoming custom and practice or your own mental flowchart (informal)?

The benefits of intentional rounding include the following.

- A more orderly ward environment whereby patients will be more comfortable and will have greater confidence that they will receive reliable care.
- Fewer random needs for support and help as care delivery is more controlled.
- A reduction in pressure ulcers and falls as tasks are scheduled rather than as and when needed.
- Rounding as an approach is flexible, and can be adapted to local circumstances, for example in reducing social isolation in patients with dementia.
- Rounding is patient-centred, and can provide a quality assurance framework for care delivery. Patients are reported to feel less isolated and know that they will be checked on regularly.

- Through audit, intentional rounding can provide evidence on what nurses do and can demonstrate the impact of care delivery.
- An increase in the morale of staff.

It is worth noting at this point that further evaluation of intentional rounding is needed to determine its effectiveness.

The limitations of intentional rounding include the following.

- Intentional rounding is task-orientated, moving away from treating patients as individuals.
- There is uncertainty as to who carries out intentional rounding, how often and for which patients.
- There is uncertainty as to the costs associated with a different model in relation to care delivery.
- There is uncertainty as to the implications for skill mix and nursing staff.

Key points to consider if you were to introduce such an approach within your own area of practice include the following.

- Rounding should be tested with care and systematically implemented, allowing for flexibility. Staff concerns should be explored as to whether it is effective, or whether it adds to workload and whether the approach should be responsive to concerns.
- Rounding should be adjusted to local needs and circumstances. A 'one size fits all' would not necessarily be the most appropriate approach. Staff should feel ownership and should be able to adapt or abandon certain elements of this different model as evidence emerges as to its effectiveness. For example, a stroke unit has patients with different needs from those on a rehabilitation unit, therefore adaptation of processes would be required.
- Strong nursing leadership, staff training and accountability may be critical to the success of rounding to support improved patient experiences of care and outcomes.
- Poorly designed checklists or excessive use of them could overcomplicate care delivery and potentially reduce efficiency.

One of the challenges to practice may be *resistance to change*. Staff may feel threatened or that the way that care is delivered is being criticised; therefore, it is vital that all staff, at every level, are involved in the process. *Clear nursing leadership*, *ongoing support* and *teamwork* are crucial to the success of intentional rounding.

By *measuring the effectiveness* of intentional rounding, necessary evidence would be generated as to whether or not it was having the desired outcome, for example in improving patient safety and satisfaction scores.

Careful consideration may need to be given to overall *cost implications* – including skill mix and nursing staff. Setting up new initiatives such as intentional rounding can be very time consuming and an intensive process for all those involved, and time does cost money. *Training* would need to be considered as a key aspect in the planning stage. Once again, due consideration would need to be given to costs associated with the necessary training. *Time to review, adapt and implement change* will also inevitably incur costs, as well as time implications, during the initial 'set-up' phase.

Sustainability and motivation are also crucial to the success of such an initiative. Once results such as the reduction of harm can be demonstrated, it is more likely that intentional rounding will become embedded into everyday care delivery and therefore sustainable. Clear nursing leadership, teamwork, ongoing support and patient satisfaction will inevitably provide staff with the motivation that they need to succeed.

Regarding whether you would need to include all patients or whether this would vary depending on patients' clinical condition or level of care required, this decision would need to be made depending on environmental circumstances. For example, a surgical unit has patients with different needs from those on a rehabilitation unit, therefore adaptation of processes would be required.

Further reading

Studer Group (2007) *Best Practices: Sacred Heart Hospital, Pensacola, Florida. Hourly Rounding Supplement*. Gulf Breeze, FL: Studer Group.

This contains useful information on the origins of intentional rounding.

Vincent, C (2010) *Patient Safety*, 2nd edition. Oxford: Wiley-Blackwell.

This is a comprehensive read on all aspects of patient safety and the practice environment.

Useful websites

http://npsa.nhs.uk/patientsafety/improvingpatientsafety/humanfactors/foresight

This website has useful information in relation to foresight training – both paper- and video-based scenarios.

http://who.int/patientsafety/implementation/checklists/background_document.pdf

This site has useful information provided by WHO regarding the Safe Childbirth Checklist programme.

www.institute.nhs.uk/quality_and_service_improvement_tools/quality_and_service_imp rovement_tools/protocol_based_care.html

On this Institute for Innovation and Improvement website you can search for protocol-based care and service improvement tools.

www.nhs.uk/NHSEngland/thenhs/healthregulators/Pages/carequalitycommission.aspx

The Care Quality Commission provides an extremely useful website offering up-to-date information on regulated health and adult social care services in England.

www.who.int/patientsafety/safesurgery/ss_checklist/en

Here you will find useful information provided by WHO regarding the Surgical Safety Checklist.

Chapter 3
Accidents and incidents – what went wrong?

NMC Standards for Pre-registration Nursing Education

This chapter will address the following competencies:

Domain 1: Professional values

4. All nurses must work in partnership with service users, carers, families, groups, communities and organisations. They must manage risk, and promote health and well-being while aiming to empower choices that promote self-care and safety.

7. All nurses must be responsible and accountable for keeping their knowledge and skills up to date through continuing professional development. They must aim to improve their performance and enhance safety and quality of care through evaluation, supervision and appraisal.

9. All nurses must appreciate the value of evidence in practice, be able to understand and appraise research, apply relevant theory and research findings to their work, and identify areas for further investigation.

Domain 2: Communication and interpersonal skills

4. All nurses must recognise when people are anxious or in distress and respond effectively, using therapeutic principles, to promote their well-being, manage personal safety and resolve conflict. They must use effective communication strategies and negotiation techniques to achieve best outcomes, respecting the dignity and human rights of all concerned. They must know when to consult a third party and how to make referrals for advocacy, mediation and arbitration.

7. All nurses must maintain accurate, clear and complete records, including the use of electronic formats, using appropriate and plain language.

8. All nurses must respect individual rights to confidentiality and keep information secure and confidential in accordance with the law and relevant ethical and regulatory frameworks, taking account of local protocols. They must also actively share personal information with others when the interests of safety and protection override the need for confidentiality.

Domain 3: Nursing practice and decision making

6. All nurses must practise safely by being aware of the correct use, limitations and hazards of common interventions, including nursing activities, treatments, and the use

continued . . .

of medical devices and equipment. The nurse must be able to evaluate their use, report any concerns promptly through appropriate channels and modify care where necessary to maintain safety. They must contribute to the collection of local and national data and formulation of policy on risks, hazards and adverse outcomes.

Domain 4: Leadership, management and team working

6. All nurses must work independently as well as in teams. They must be able to take the lead in co-ordinating, delegating and supervising care safely, managing risk and remaining accountable for the care given.

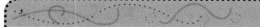

NMC Essential Skills Clusters

This chapter will address the following ESCs:

Cluster: Care, compassion and communication

1. As partners in the care process, people can trust a newly registered graduate nurse to provide collaborative care based on the highest standards, knowledge and competence.

By entry to the register:

8. Demonstrates clinical confidence through sound knowledge, skills and understanding relevant to field.
9. Is self aware and self-confident, knows own limitations and is able to take appropriate action.

Cluster: Organisational aspects of care

9. People can trust the newly registered graduate to treat them as partners and work with them to make a holistic and systematic assessment of their needs; to develop a personalised plan that is based on mutual understanding and respect for their individual situation promoting health and well-being, minimising risk of harm and promoting their safety at all times.
12. People can trust the newly registered graduate nurse to respond to their feedback and a wide range of other sources to learn, develop and improve services.
17. People can trust the newly registered graduate to work safely under pressure and maintain the safety of the service users at all times.
18. People can trust the newly registered graduate nurse to enhance the safety of service users and identify and actively manage risk and uncertainty in relation to people, the environment, self and others.

By entry to the register:

9. Reflects on and learns from safety incidents as an autonomous individual and as a team member and contributes to team learning.
11. Assesses and implements measures to manage, reduce or remove risk that could be detrimental to people, self and others.
14. Works within policies to protect self and others in all care settings including the home care setting.

Introduction

NEWS HEADLINE – The Department of Health has set a target to deliver 'harm-free care' to 95 per cent of patients, by 2012.

The purpose of this chapter will be to explore some of the key features that can contribute to mistakes and how mistakes can lead to patient harm. First, we will focus upon approaches, tools and models, which can be used to identify the cause of a problem that could harm a patient. Root cause analysis (RCA), first established by the National Center for Patient Safety in the US Department of Veterans Affairs, and the **London Protocol** (Taylor-Adams and Vincent, 2004) will be introduced with working examples of how each tool can be applied to practice, and how through action planning the likelihood of the same or similar mistake happening again can be greatly reduced. A further important theme of this chapter will be incident reporting and the value of learning from reporting. We will take into account some of the barriers to reporting that we know exist. Towards the end of the chapter **system failure** and individual blame will be discussed in light of an incident that could have caused, or did cause, harm to a patient and how the development of the **Incident Decision Tree** has helped managers to take a fair and consistent approach towards staff rather than that of disciplinary action or suspension. Practical examples and case studies from an organisational and individual point of view illustrate applications of key principles relating to the patient safety agenda in different clinical contexts.

Root cause analysis

Root cause analysis (RCA) is a systematic, problem-solving approach that aims to identify the true cause of a problem and the actions necessary to ensure that the problem will not happen again. RCA is a reactive method of highlighting the problem and then providing a solution; it is not a single method and there are many different tools and processes for performing RCA. It is not always people at the root cause of the problem; more often than not it is procedures and processes, or the lack of them. It is worth noting that there may be several potential root causes for any one problem. One strategy to make sure all causes have been identified is the '**five whys**' technique. This technique is simple and easy to learn and will very quickly help to identify the root cause of a problem. By repeatedly asking the question 'why?' five times you can peel away the layers of a problem, rather like taking off layers of clothing on a hot, sunny day. The reason for a problem can often lead to another question and so on. RCA originated in the field of engineering, but more recently the value of RCA has been recognised in healthcare. This was driven by the fact that healthcare delivery has become increasingly complex and the number of incidents or mistakes that have put patients at risk from harm has increased (WHO, 2004a).

Case study

Mr James Smith is a 65-year-old man who was admitted to hospital for various investigations, including a barium swallow (meal). Mr Smith has been nil by mouth overnight in preparation for this procedure. Karen is a newly appointed band 5 staff nurse on the ward and is very keen to fit into the well-established team. Karen receives a call from the radiology department asking her to prepare Mr James Smith for his barium swallow as a time slot has become available to perform the procedure. Karen quickly and efficiently helps Mr Smith into his gown, explaining that a time for his procedure has been allocated.

Meanwhile Sally, the healthcare assistant, is preparing Mr James Smith, a 68-year-old gentleman, for transfer to another ward for rehabilitation. Sally has carefully packed all Mr Smith's belongings, including his notes, drug kardex and X-rays ready for transfer. The porter arrives to take Mr Smith to the ward. Sally accompanies Mr Smith, taking with her all of Mr Smith's belongings and documentation.

A second porter arrives on the ward to take Mr James Smith to radiology for his barium swallow. Karen goes to the office to collect notes and previous X-rays for Mr Smith; she is unable to find them and spends valuable time looking for them. The porter starts to get anxious as 20 minutes later the notes and X-rays have not been found. Karen then realises what has happened and that Sally has taken the wrong notes, drug kardex and X-rays to the rehabilitation ward. By the time Karen contacts Sally and explains the situation Mr James Smith has missed his allocated time slot in radiology. The radiology department cannot accommodate Mr Smith until the next day. Mr Smith is upset as he has been nil by mouth for the procedure. Karen apologises to Mr Smith for the mistake. Karen finishes her shift and begins to worry that she may be blamed for what has happened.

What we can see in this case study involving two patients with the same name is that coincidences can create confusion and ultimately lead to mistakes. The most important aspect of analysing an error or mistake is to discover what happened and how to prevent it from happening again. RCA would be just one approach that could be used and focuses on the system or process, not the individual. An assumption is made that the mistake is a system failure. System failure is covered more thoroughly in Chapter 7.

Activity 3.1   *Reflection*

Take some time to think about the implications of the case study.

- What might this mean for the patient who did not undergo the procedure?
- What implications might this have for Karen in the long term?
- How are other members of staff likely to feel about the situation?
- Other than an apology, could Karen have considered doing anything else?
- Consider the outcome if, for example, Mr James Smith (aged 65), received Mr James Smith's (aged 68) medications.

Outline answers and thoughts are provided at the end of the chapter.

If we consider applying the 'five whys' technique to the case study we may be able to identify the problem and then provide a solution.

Question 1: Why did Mr James Smith, aged 65, miss his appointment for a barium swallow?

Answer: Karen, the staff nurse, was unable to find his notes and previous X-rays.

Question 2: Why was Karen unable to find the notes and X-rays belonging to Mr James Smith?

Answer: There were two patients on the ward with exactly the same name. Mr James Smith, aged 68, was transferred to the rehabilitation ward with the other patient's notes, drug kardex and X-rays.

Question 3: Why did this situation arise?

Answer: There were no distinguishing features between the two sets of notes, even though the patients had the same name.

Question 4: Why was there no way of making a distinction between the notes?

Answer: There was no strategy, policy or procedure in place for patients who were admitted to the ward with the same or very similar names.

Question 5: Why was there no system in place?

Answer: This type of situation had never happened before on the ward.

Solution to the problem using root cause analysis

Although this may seem like a very simple example, it allows you to consider the principles of applying the 'five whys' technique to a practice situation. This type of error has occurred and still does, even without the coincidence depicted in the case study. By adopting a team approach to the example given in the case study, effective meaningful changes could be made so that the same mistake did not happen again. It is up to the entire team to make a safe and harm-free environment in which to care for patients. If the same situation happens again, where two patients have the same or similar names, a clear strategy or protocol has to be developed. This reduces the likelihood of a mistake occurring again.

An alternative approach that you might like to consider, depending on your practice area, is that of significant event analysis (SEA). The introduction and development of this technique came from the work of two general practitioners (GPs), Mike Pringle and Colin Bradley. SEA is a relatively new and qualitative method of clinical audit that is concerned with looking at individual events that have been identified by a member of the healthcare team. The idea is that by reflecting on events and learning from mistakes the quality and safety of the care that is delivered to patients will be improved. This approach is favoured in primary care settings and, although different, it does in fact have some similarities to RCA. GPs are now required to provide evidence that they are using SEA as part of their contracts.

Common types of significant events that occur in primary care settings are not so different from mistakes that can happen in the acute hospital setting. Some of those mistakes can include prescribing errors, failure to deal with an emergency call and confusion in relation to patients with the same name.

SEA involves working as a team to review events and act on:

- what happened;
- why it happened;
- what has been learned;
- what has been changed.

The London Protocol

The London Protocol is a model that uses RCA principles. The London Protocol outlines a process where an error or a mistake can be looked into and considered, and suggestions made to prevent the same mistake from happening again. It is a simple model that takes a team of healthcare professionals, or an individual, through the chain of events leading up to the mistake or error.

The steps in the Protocol's process are as follows:

- acknowledging that a mistake or error has happened and then making a decision to look into it;
- selecting the people (or person) who need to be involved in the process;
- gathering information and facts in relation to the mistake;
- finding out the order in which events occurred leading up to the error or mistake;

- identifying the care delivery problems;
- identifying what caused the care delivery problems;
- making recommendations and action plans.

Solution to the problem using the London Protocol

If we consider applying the London Protocol to the case study involving two patients with the same name (page 43), once again we may be able to identify the problem and then provide a solution.

- Acknowledging that a mistake or error has happened and then making a decision to look into it.

Karen has acknowledged that a mistake has been made and she has apologised to Mr Smith. Karen feels that, in some way, she was to blame for what happened and when she returns to duty the next day she decides to look into the mistake that was made.

- Selecting the people (or person) who need to be involved in the process.

Karen considers involving Sally in the process as she feels that they can both learn from the mistake. Together Karen and Sally might be able to suggest some measure that could be put in place to prevent a similar mistake.

- Gathering information and facts in relation to the mistake.

It does not take Karen and Sally very long to gather the information and facts they need in relation to the mistake. They both realise that two patients on the same ward had exactly the same name and there was no quick way of distinguishing between the two sets of notes.

- Finding out the order in which events occurred leading up to the error or mistake.

Systematically, Karen and Sally recall the sequence of events leading up to the realisation of the mistake.

At 0840 – Karen received a call from radiology requesting that Mr James Smith (aged 65) be prepared for his barium meal at 1000.

At 0850 – Karen prepares Mr James Smith (aged 65) for his barium meal. Sally is packing up Mr James Smith's (aged 68) belongings, ready for transfer to the rehabilitation ward. Mr James Smith (aged 68) was in the bathroom having a shave.

At 0930 – The first porter arrives to transfer Mr James Smith (aged 68) to the rehabilitation ward. Sally remembers feeling flustered as Mr James Smith (aged 68) was still in the bathroom. All his belongings were packed and ready to go to the rehabilitation ward but Mr James Smith (aged 68) could not find any clean pyjamas. Sally quickly got them out of his packed belongings and helped him to put them on.

At 0945 – The porter was getting agitated as he had a number of other patients to transfer that morning. Once Mr James Smith (aged 68) was settled into the wheelchair they left the ward. Sally suddenly remembered his notes and hurried into the office to collect them. It was at this point that the incorrect notes were taken.

At 0950 – The second porter arrives to collect Mr James Smith (aged 65) for his investigation. Karen was at that point talking to a relative on the telephone.

At 1000 – Karen finished the call and assisted Mr James Smith into a wheelchair ready to be taken to radiology. Karen looked for his notes but could only find those belonging to Mr James Smith (aged 68). Twenty minutes later Karen realised the mistake and by the time Sally came back with the other set of notes it was 1035 and the time slot in radiology had been missed.

- Identifying the care delivery problems.

Mr James Smith (aged 65) had missed a very important investigation and, although he did not suffer direct harm, he had been unable to eat breakfast because of being nil by mouth. Karen also realised that there would be a delay in Mr Smith receiving a definite diagnosis and subsequently this could lead to a delay in treatment (active failure – to understand further, please refer to Chapter 7).

- Identifying what caused the care delivery problems.

There were no distinguishing features between the two sets of notes, even though the patients had the same name.

- Making recommendations and action plans.

Karen and Sally approached the ward manager and recommended that there should be a procedure in place for patients who were admitted to the ward with the same or very similar names. Karen asked the ward manager if she could take responsibility for the action plan as she felt it was within her capabilities as a band 5 staff nurse.

Again, we have considered the same very simple example but this time it allows you to consider the principles of applying a different model based on the London Protocol to a practice situation.

From the RCA and London Protocol examples you will by now have recognised that the outcome for the practice area was the same. An agreed action plan or protocol could easily be developed, reducing the likelihood of the same mistake occurring again.

Activity 3.2   *Evidence-based practice and research*

- Try to find out if there are any strategies, protocols or procedures in place to distinguish between two patients with the same or similar names if admitted to your practice area.
- You might also like to consider something similar for another practice area in which you have worked, so that you can get an overview of different strategies or solutions to the same problem.

Answers will be based on your own observations, but some ideas have been suggested at the end of the chapter.

Ways to learn from mistakes or errors

Incident reporting

In simple terms an error or mistake usually happens when someone is trying to do the right thing, but actually does the wrong thing.

When we look closely at mistakes we can often find out what happened by using models such as RCA. We can come up with ideas, protocols or checklists to prevent mistakes from occurring again. What we must also think about is the learning that needs to take place. It is believed that, by reporting mistakes that could have caused ('near miss') or did cause harm to the patient, valuable learning can take place in order to reduce the likelihood of a similar occurrence happening in the future.

Incident reporting is a term that is widely acknowledged, accepted and carried out in the acute practice area. Recognising the value of incident reporting is perhaps less apparent in other practice settings, for example primary care practice areas. It is generally known that incidents are underreported, often because those who do report incidents are blamed for their involvement. It is only natural that you would avoid reporting a mistake that has been made if you are to be blamed for that mistake. By not reporting mistakes opportunities for learning are missed and it is highly likely that the same mistake will be made again.

Scenario

Imagine that you are a student on the ward where Karen and Sally work. You finish your shift at the same time as Karen. While you are getting ready to go home Karen confides in you that she is worried that, when the ward manager finds out about Mr James Smith missing his investigation due to the confusion over notes, she will be blamed.

- *Do you feel that Karen has cause to be concerned?*
- *What do you think may contribute to Karen feeling this way?*
- *Do you feel that Karen should have reported the mistake?*
- *Do you feel that you could report the mistake even though you were only a witness?*

This scenario, at first glance, may not really seem that important, particularly as Mr Smith came to no visible harm. Karen might feel that she will be blamed as it is well recognised that staff are less likely to report errors or raise safety concerns if they are punished or blamed. As within the case study, most mistakes and errors are due to a weakness in the system, which then affects the performance of the individual within the system. If you are a witness to a mistake you are still able to report that mistake, although you might then feel that you are being disloyal. It is important to note that occasion might arise where you have a duty of care and a professional obligation to report a mistake that has been made.

Barriers to learning from mistakes

All too often when something goes wrong in healthcare those in charge will overemphasise the contributions of one or two individuals and pin the blame for the error or mistake on them. While blame may be appropriate in certain circumstances, it should not be the starting point. Barriers to learning from an error or a mistake include a blame culture that often focuses too much on the actions of individuals rather than the background to such events.

A culture of blame may contribute to Karen feeling the way she does and as a result this can drive reporting underground. This will prevent us from learning what makes things safer. Karen should have reported the mistake so that learning can take place and systems can be set up to reduce the likelihood of the same or similar mistakes from happening again. For Karen to feel comfortable enough to report the mistake, the organisation in which she works needs to make a clear commitment to staff that they fully support an open and fair reporting culture. When a mistake is made, staff should feel able to be honest and open and know that they will be treated fairly. By actively encouraging a reporting culture failures within the system can be identified and improved, rather than seeking to blame specific individuals. If you had been a witness to the mistake made by Karen and Sally and they decided not to report the mistake it would inevitably put you in a very difficult position. If the culture within the organisation was supportive, open and fair, you might feel better able to report the mistake.

The National Patient Safety Agency (NPSA, 2011a) very clearly encourages the reporting of *all patient safety incidents*. This includes:

- incidents in which you have been involved;
- incidents that you may have witnessed;
- incidents that caused no harm or minimal harm;
- incidents with a more serious outcome;
- prevented patient safety incidents (known as 'near misses').

By now there should be no doubt in your mind as to whether or not the incident involving two patients with the same name should have been reported. If you are still uncertain apply the reporting criteria to the case study.

Activity 3.3   *Critical thinking*

Take a moment to reflect on the case study involving two patients with the same name (page 43). We have established that the incident should have been reported. Even though the patient did not come to any direct harm this type of incident could have been classed as a 'near misss'. The NPSA recommends and actively encourages all incidents, including 'near misses' to be reported. Imagine if you are the nurse in Karen's position and then write down your answers to the following questions. You might find it useful to read through the case study again.

- Would you know how to report an incident in your practice area?
- Do you feel that your practice area actively encourages incident reporting?

continued . . .

- Would you feel confident enough to report an incident or 'near miss'?
- Is there a policy relating to incident reporting in your practice area?

As this activity is for you to review your own experience, no answer is provided, but you might find it useful to discuss your responses and any related development needs with your clinical mentor.

The role of the National Reporting and Learning System

The National Patient Safety Agency (NPSA) was established in 2001 to facilitate and coordinate changes in culture and practice across the NHS, with the aim of promoting and improving patient safety. One of its key roles was to create a National Reporting and Learning System (NRLS). The function of the NRLS is twofold: to capture incidents that could or do lead to harm and to learn from them.

On 1 June 2012 the key functions and expertise for patient safety developed by the NPSA transferred to the NHS Commissioning Board Special Health Authority, now NHS England, which harnessed the power of the NRLS. The NRLS is the world's most comprehensive database for the collection of patient safety information. All healthcare organisations should continue to report incidents to the NRLS so that the root cause can be tackled and learning from incidents can take place. The ultimate goal is to reduce the likelihood of harm to patients no matter where care is delivered.

Promoting effective reporting

In 2001 the Kennedy Report was published following the Bristol Royal Infirmary Inquiry (BRI, 2001). One of the key recommendations was that every effort should be made to create an open and non-punitive (no blame) environment in the NHS in which it is safe to report and admit incidents. The Government has since made it very clear that being open and fair must be a top priority in healthcare.

The Incident Decision Tree

In organisations with a culture of safety such as the NHS, creating an environment that is free from blame or punishment is a work in progress. The Incident Decision Tree was developed by the NPSA in 2003, which aimed to help the NHS move away from a culture of blame and punishment to that of finding out the cause of why something went wrong. The overall goal is to promote fair and consistent treatment of staff within and between healthcare organisations.

The Incident Decision Tree is based on an algorithm that allows managers to consider alternatives to suspending or disciplining staff who might have been involved in an event or mistake that has caused harm. The Incident Decision Tree aims to encourage open and transparent reporting in a fair and consistent way. In Figure 3.1 you will see four key questions that need to be answered. Possible reasons for the individual's action are reviewed and the most likely

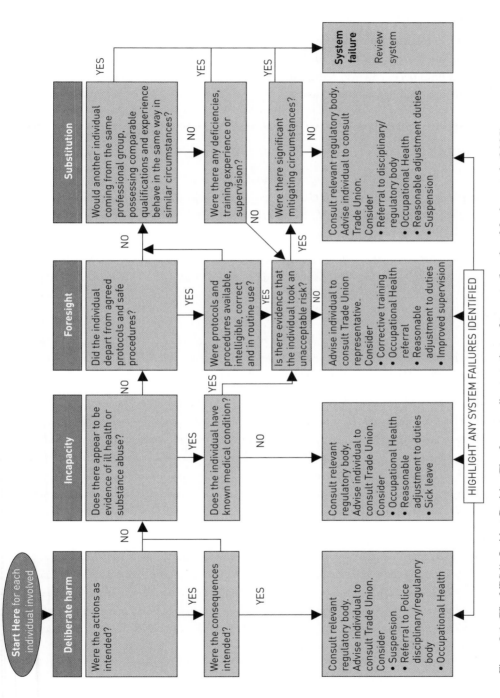

Figure 3.1: The NPSA's Incident Decision Tree for responding to patient safety events (based on Meadows et al., 2005)

explanation identified. We will apply the Incident Decision Tree to a practical example later in the chapter. This will help you to understand that there are alternatives to punishment and blame.

As we already know, system failures are often the root cause of a mistake. It is worth noting that the Incident Decision Tree complements the RCA model. The most common response to a more serious mistake is to suspend and then discipline the staff involved. This can be a very unfair approach and often detracts from finding out what caused the system or systems to fail. Suspending key employees can also reduce the quality of care that a patient can expect to receive, as those people are unable to come to work.

Case study

Jacqueline, a 32-year-old professional dancer, was admitted to the day unit for a right knee arthroscopy and meniscectomy under general anaesthetic. Mr Green, her consultant orthopaedic surgeon, had obtained consent from Jacqueline for the procedure earlier that morning. He had also marked her right knee with a black 'X' prior to the operation, as per limb surgery protocol.

Jacqueline was asked to prepare herself for the operation by having a shower and putting on a hospital gown ready to go to the operating theatre. When Jacqueline was drying herself after the shower she noticed that the black 'X' had faded, but was still slightly visible. The porter arrived for Jacqueline and she was taken to theatre.

All appropriate checklists were completed in the reception bay of theatre, including a check of the limb to be operated on. Jacqueline confirmed that she had signed the consent form and that it was the right knee that required surgery. Staff Nurse Francis took her to the anaesthetic room.

Meanwhile, in the adjacent theatre, Mr Green was experiencing a problem with some equipment while performing a total hip replacement. He was conscious of the time and that Jacqueline was waiting in the anaesthetic room. Mr Green knew that his senior registrar was capable of performing the arthroscopy and meniscectomy and asked him if he could start Jacqueline's surgery. The theatre manager was trying to resolve the issue with the equipment, realising that he was supposed to be in the adjacent theatre with the senior registrar. The equipment failure would require a replacement part but the spare had been used during an earlier procedure and was waiting to be sterilised.

Staff Nurse Davis had been qualified for a year but was new to the operating department. Her previous job had been working in the outpatients department but this had only been a temporary contract. Staff Nurse Davis was working as the circulating nurse in the theatre where Jacqueline was to have her surgery. She was unfamiliar with the 'time out' surgical checklist and some important checks were unintentionally missed out (see page 26 on the WHO's Surgical Safety Checklist). While Staff Nurse Davis was waiting for the senior registrar to 'scrub up', she put Jacqueline's X-ray up on to the viewing screen. In doing so she placed the X-ray the wrong way round so that the right knee now appeared to be the left knee.

Jacqueline was brought into the operating theatre from the anaesthetic room, by which time the theatre manager was scrubbing up in readiness to assist the senior registrar. The senior registrar quickly glanced at the X-ray and started to prepare Jacqueline's left knee for surgery. He could not see any black 'X' on either knee and

continued . . .

> *thought to himself that this was rather remiss of Mr Green. The theatre manager quickly joined the senior registrar but his thoughts were very much on the equipment problem in the adjacent theatre. The surgery went ahead on Jacqueline's left knee.*
>
> *It was when Jacqueline woke up in the recovery area that she realised something must have gone wrong, as it was her left knee that was bandaged and not her right knee. Mr Green was informed of the error. At this point Jacqueline was furious, very tearful and uncertain as to her future as a professional dancer.*

If we review the case study involving Jacqueline it is very easy to see that it was a sequence of events that led up to the mistake been made. Human error is routinely blamed for events such as these. People who are not directly involved in the event are very quick to make judgements and allocate blame, but what this does is hide a more complex truth.

The identification of an obvious departure from good practice is usually only the very first step of an investigation. Closer scrutiny usually reveals a series of events and departures from good practice, influenced by the working environment and the wider organisational context. No one person is necessarily responsible or to blame for the outcome. What we do know through reporting such incidents as highlighted within the case study is that it is not unusual for there to be a complex chain of events leading up to a negative outcome (see Chapter 7, page 119, on the 'Swiss cheese' model). The root cause analysis of an incident like Jacqueline's may lie in a number of interlocking factors, such as poor communication within a team, supervision problems, excessive workload and training deficiencies.

The following scenario gives an example of how easy it is to want to blame someone for harm that has been unintentionally caused.

Scenario

Imagine that you are Jacqueline's partner and you have come in to visit Jacqueline following her surgery. When you arrive on the ward you can see Jacqueline lying on the bed. You notice that she has been crying, as her eyes are red and blotchy. You hurry towards Jacqueline, as you are concerned. Jacqueline sobs, 'They have operated on the wrong knee. My career is over!'

What are your immediate thoughts and feelings:

1. *disbelief and anger?*
2. *upset and concern for Jacqueline's future?*
3. *wanting to blame someone for what has happened?*
4. *wanting an explanation of how this type of incident could have possibly happened?*
5. *that whoever is responsible for such a mistake should never be allowed to work again?*
6. *all of the above?*

The chances are that your immediate thoughts and feelings in response to the scenario would be 'all of the above'.

Activity 3.4	*Decision making*

If you take more time to consider response 3 from the scenario that involves Jacqueline's partner, who do you think could or possibly should be to blame:

- Mr Green (orthopaedic consultant);
- the senior registrar;
- the theatre manager;
- Staff Nurse Francis;
- Staff Nurse Davis?

As this activity is based on your own thoughts, there is no answer at the end of the chapter.

If all the people involved in Jacqueline's operation were to be suspended from duty and then disciplined, this would undoubtedly have an impact on the quality of care for other patients, as those people would not be allowed to come to work. The Incident Decision Tree is a tool that can help managers decide on what action to take with staff who have been involved in an incident that has caused harm to a patient. The tool is based on a flowchart, which guides the user through a series of structured questions about the individual's actions, motives and behaviours at the time of the incident. The responses to these questions lead to suggestions for appropriate management action. The tool is applied to each individual involved.

The Incident Decision Tree can help managers:

- consider other possible measures to be taken;
- decide whether it is necessary to suspend staff from duty following an incident that has resulted in harm to the patient;
- consider alternative duties rather than suspension.

Application of the Incident Decision Tree to practice

If we consider applying the principles of the Incident Decision Tree to Staff Nurse Davis from the case study we might be able to come up with an action plan for her. Remember that Staff Nurse Davis was new to the operating department environment. She had previously worked in an outpatient department but this was only a temporary contract and she wanted permanent employment. Staff Nurse Davis did not fully understand the relevance of the 'time out' surgical checklist and some important checks were unintentionally missed. She was also responsible for placing the X-ray on the viewing screen, but it was the wrong way round so the right knee looked like the left knee.

See Figure 3.1 (page 51), as we will need to use the flowchart to help us to make a decision.

What we now need to consider are the questions identified along the top row of the flowchart and apply them to what we know about Staff Nurse Davis. Note the arrow 'Start Here'.

Question 1

Deliberate harm test

Were the actions as intended?

What we need to think about is whether or not Staff Nurse Davis set out to cause harm to Jacqueline. In the majority of cases where a patient has been harmed, the individual has the patient's well-being at heart and the outcome for the patient was by no means intended. We can now state that Staff Nurse Davis's actions were as intended, but the outcome was indeed not. Staff Nurse Davis did not intentionally set out to cause harm to Jacqueline. As the answer to question 1 is no, we then move across to:

Question 2

Incapacity test

Does there appear to be evidence of ill health or substance abuse?

As we have decided that Staff Nurse Davis did not intend to harm Jacqueline, we now need to consider Staff Nurse Davis's health. The incapacity test helps to identify whether ill health or substance abuse, including self-medicating, caused or contributed to the incident. From what we know from the case study and Staff Nurse Davis's involvement it would seem reasonable to think that she was not suffering from ill health or working while under the influence of drugs or alcohol. As the answer to question 2 is no, we then move across to:

Question 3

Foresight test

Did the individual depart from agreed protocols or safe procedures?

We have now decided that Staff Nurse Davis did not intend to harm Jacqueline and that incapacity due to ill health or substance abuse has been ruled out, so we move along the flowchart. The foresight test considers whether protocols and safe practices were adhered to. We know that Staff Nurse Davis was new to the operating department and she was uncertain as to the relevance of the 'time out' surgical checklist. We can now state that Staff Nurse Davis did not follow the protocol due to her lack of training, as she was new to the department. There has been a protocol violation and departure from best practice (see Chapter 2, pages 23–4, for protocol violation). It is worth noting at this point that the majority of situations that lead to harm involve protocol violation or departure from best practice. As the answer to question 3 is yes, we then move down the flowchart. We now need to consider:

Were the protocols and safe procedures available, workable, intelligible, correct and in routine use?

We know that the 'time out' surgical checklist was in use, but we also know that Staff Nurse Davis was unfamiliar with the process and unintentionally missed out some important checks. We would also need to consider the circumstances as to why Nurse Davis did not adhere to the checklist. Remember that Dr Green was busy in the adjacent theatre; there were issues with equipment, the theatre manager was delayed trying to arrange alternative equipment and the senior registrar was instructed to carry out Jacqueline's operation. Staff Nurse Davis, who was a new member of staff, was left in a position where she was working without direct supervision and was unfamiliar with systems and processes. The situation was chaotic and it could be that Staff Nurse Davis was under extreme pressure and had little time to think about the consequences, so to some extent it is easy to see why the incident occurred. The answer to this particular question is yes, so once again we move down the flowchart. We now need to ask ourselves:

Is there evidence that the individual took an unacceptable risk?

What we now must think about is whether or not Staff Nurse Davis was taking a risk that could be considered unreasonable. We would need to look at Staff Nurse Davis's motivation and circumstances rather than the potential consequences of her actions. Staff Nurse Davis was new to the department, working without support or supervision. The circumstances in which she was working happened to be chaotic for several reasons. Staff Nurse Davis did deviate from policy but did not intentionally set out to harm Jacqueline. The answer to the question is no, so we move down the flowchart one last time.

Practical alternative to suspension

After reviewing Staff Nurse Davis's involvement in the incident with Jacqueline, an alternative to suspension could be considered. The action plan might include:

* placing restrictions on Staff Nurse Davis's practice;
* moving Staff Nurse Davis to another work area;
* placing Staff Nurse Davis under more intense supervision;
* corrective training.

Suspension or disciplinary action might not necessarily be the only outcome for an individual involved in an incident that caused harm to a patient. By applying the Incident Decision Tree flowchart to a practice situation, alternatives can be considered in relation to that individual.

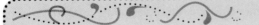

Chapter summary

This chapter attempted to explain that the majority of incidents that can and do cause harm to patients are due to system failures rather than individuals. We have looked very closely at root cause analysis and the application of such an approach to the practice area. You have also been given the opportunity to consider the value of reporting incidents that occur in practice. You now have some ideas, tools and methods on which you can build your own knowledge base and develop the necessary skills to be able to contribute to the patient safety agenda, no matter where you practise.

Activities: brief outline answers

Activity 3.1: Reflection (page 44)

The patient missed a very important investigation and, although he did not suffer direct harm, he had been unable to eat breakfast because of being nil by mouth. There would be a delay in Mr Smith receiving a definite diagnosis and subsequently this could lead to a delay in treatment (active failure – to understand further, please refer to Chapter 7).

Karen may well feel a loss of confidence in her own abilities. As Karen is newly qualified she may be finding the transition from a student nurse to being a registrant difficult. She may feel that this incident may threaten her career prospects. Karen may also feel that other members of the team could consider her to be incompetent within her new role and that they want to blame her for the mistake. These feelings could have a lasting effect on Karen.

Other staff may feel that this is a small mistake that could have happened to anyone under the circumstances. There was no lasting harm to Mr Smith and therefore nothing to be concerned about. Some staff members may view this situation very differently and may want to blame or punish Karen for the mistake. Mr Smith has been inconvenienced and there will be a delay in his diagnosis, so someone needs to take responsibility for the mistake.

Karen could have considered reporting this mistake, for example through completing an incident report. This may be referred to as an IR1 or datix depending on your practice area.

Mistakes in relation to a patient receiving another patient's medication do happen and the consequences may be unpredictable. The outcome would very much depend on the medication. If, for example, it was a unit of blood, the outcome could be very serious or even fatal. Alternatively, if it was a gram of paracetamol, the likelihood is that it would have few or no consequences. What we would need to recognise is the fact that a mistake has been made and we would then need to report the incident. Learning from our mistakes is very important.

Activity 3.2: Evidence-based practice and research (page 47)

It could be that some practice areas have a very distinct 'name alert' protocol, while other practice areas may approach the situation by attaching flags in the two sets of notes highlighting the fact that patients have the same or similar names. A note may be made above the patient's bedhead alerting everyone to the fact that two patients have the same or similar names.

Further reading

Taylor-Adams, S and Vincent, C (2004) *Systems Analysis of Clinical Incidents – The London Protocol.* London: Clinical Safety Research Unit, Imperial College London.

This document will provide the reader with a comprehensive overview of the London Protocol and the application of principles to practice. The London Protocol is a refined and developed approach originating from the 'Protocol for the Investigation and Analysis of Clinical Incidents'. The London Protocol goes beyond the fault and blame culture to that of investigation and analysis. A very interesting and thought-provoking read.

It can also be found at: www1.imperial.ac.uk/resources/C85B6574-7E28-4BE6-BE61-E94C3F6243CE/londonprotocol_e.pdf

Useful websites

http://gptraining.dundee.ac.uk/docs/2011/NES%20SEA%20Guide%20FinalVersion%20 2011.pdf

This website provides guidance on significant event analysis. It highlights the purpose and background and offers working examples as well as guidance on how to apply the principles of SEA to practice. Further reading and references are also detailed, including the work of Mike Pringle and Colin Bradley.

www.npsa.nhs.uk

This link will take you to the home page of the National Patient Safety Agency. The website will provide current information on patient safety, incident reporting and alerts and tools. It might be useful to visit this website prior to an interview, as patient safety incident reports are available for most Trusts in England and Wales, including primary care, mental health and learning disabilities.

www.nrls.npsa.nhs.uk/resources/?EntryId45=59900

This link provides brief information on the Incident Decision Tree. Although it may not be a comprehensive link, the information is concise and appropriate.

www.patientsafety.va.gov

This patient safety link will guide you to the National Center for Patient Safety (NCPS), which was first established in 1999. The Department of Veterans Affairs was developed to provide a safety culture throughout the Veterans Health Administration. Its goal is to reduce and prevent harm occurring to patients as a result of their care. Root cause analysis (RCA) as a method of problem solving was first established within the NCPS. Although first established in 1999, the website provides useful information in relation to the safety agenda. As this department is based in the United States it is worth noting that some policies and practices may differ from those provided in the UK.

www.who.int/patientsafety/worldalliance/en

This link provides comprehensive information in relation to the World Health Organization World Alliance for Patient Safety. Launched on 27 October 2004, with the aim that heads of agencies, health policy makers, representatives of patients' groups and the World Health Organization could come together and work collectively to advance the patient safety agenda of 'First do no harm', and reduce the far-reaching consequences of events that could harm patients. By typing 'root cause analysis' into the search box practical examples will be provided, detailing the impact RCA can have on delivering safer care. In some cases global, regional and national statistics and examples are given.

Chapter 4
Medicine administration and safety

continued . . .

4. All nurses must recognise when people are anxious or in distress and respond effectively, using therapeutic principles, to promote their well-being, manage personal safety and resolve conflict. They must use effective communication strategies and negotiation techniques to achieve best outcomes, respecting the dignity and human rights of all concerned. They must know when to consult a third party and how to make referrals for advocacy, mediation and arbitration.

7. All nurses must maintain accurate, clear and complete records, including the use of electronic formats, using appropriate and plain language.

8. All nurses must respect individual rights to confidentiality and keep information secure and confidential in accordance with the law and relevant ethical and regulatory frameworks, taking account of local protocols. They must also actively share personal information with others when the interests of safety and protection override the need for confidentiality.

Domain 3: Nursing practice and decision making

6. All nurses must practise safely by being aware of the correct use, limitations and hazards of common interventions, including nursing activities, treatments, and the use of medical devices and equipment. The nurse must be able to evaluate their use, report any concerns promptly through appropriate channels and modify care where necessary to maintain safety. They must contribute to the collection of local and national data and formulation of policy on risks, hazards and adverse outcomes.

Domain 4: Leadership, management and team working

6. All nurses must work independently as well as in teams. They must be able to take the lead in co-ordinating, delegating and supervising care safely, managing risk and remaining accountable for the care given.

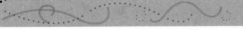

NMC Essential Skills Clusters

This chapter will address the following ESCs:

Cluster: Care, compassion and communication

2. People can trust the newly registered graduate nurse to engage in person centred care empowering people to make choices about how their needs are met when they are unable to meet them for themselves.

By entry to the register:

11. Uses strategies to manage situations where a person's wishes conflict with nursing interventions necessary for the person's safety.

Cluster: Organisational aspects of care

9. People can trust the newly registered graduate to treat them as partners and work with them to make a holistic and systematic assessment of their needs; to develop a personalised plan that is based on mutual understanding and respect for their individual

continued . . .

situation promoting health and well-being, minimising risk of harm and promoting their safety at all times.

10. People can trust the newly registered graduate nurse to deliver nursing interventions and evaluate their effectiveness against the agreed assessment and care plan.

17. People can trust the newly registered graduate nurse to work safely under pressure and maintain the safety of the service users at all times.

18. People can trust the newly registered graduate nurse to enhance the safety of service users and identify and actively manage risk and uncertainty in relation to people, the environment, self and others.

By entry to the register:

9. Reflects on and learns from safety incidents as an autonomous individual and as a team member and contributes to team learning.

10. Participates in clinical audit to improve the safety of service users.

11. Assesses and implements measures to manage, reduce or remove risk that could be detrimental to people, self and others.

12. Assesses, evaluates and interprets risk indicators and balances risks against benefits taking account of the level of risk people are prepared to take.

14. Works within policies to protect self and others in all care settings including the home care setting.

Cluster: Medicines management

36. People can trust the newly registered graduate nurse to enhance safe and effective practice in medicines management through comprehensive knowledge of medicines, their actions, risks and benefits.

By entry to the register:

4. Safely manages drug administration and monitors effects.

5. Reports adverse incidents and near misses.

38. People can trust the newly registered graduate nurse to administer medicines safely and in a timely manner, including controlled drugs.

By entry to the register:

4. Safely and effectively administers and, where necessary, prepares medicines via routes and methods commonly used and maintains accurate records.

5. Supervises and teaches others to do the same.

6. Understands the legal requirements.

39. People can trust the newly registered graduate nurse to keep and maintain accurate records using information technology, where appropriate, within a multi-disciplinary framework as a leader and as part of a team and in a variety of care settings including at home.

By entry to the register:

2. Effectively keeps records of medication administered and omitted, in a variety of care settings, including controlled drugs and ensures others do the same.

continued . . .

41. People can trust the newly registered graduate nurse to use and evaluate up-to-date information on medicines management and work within national and local policy guidelines.

By entry to the register:
2. Works within national and local policies and ensures others do the same.

Chapter aims

After reading this chapter, you will be able to:

* identify the safety risks associated with the administration of medicines;
* understand why medicines administration can sometimes result in an error being made;
* understand the nurse's role in relation to safe administration of medicines;
* understand the guiding policies and standards that are in place to promote safe administration of medicine.

Introduction

Case study

The following registered nurses are awaiting a decision following a 'fitness to practise' hearing at the NMC.

Lorraine: *Concerns were raised by the acute Trust who employed her that, as a band 5 registered nurse, she failed to demonstrate the standards of knowledge, skill and judgement required to practise without supervision. On specific dates she attempted to measure 0.25mg of a liquid medicine in a 10ml syringe. She failed to demonstrate knowledge relating to morphine sulphate on six occasions when questioned, despite attending a training and development update.*

Joseph: *Joseph is a band 5 registered nurse who failed to sign for the medication he administered on five occasions. He also left the medicine cabinet unlocked on the children's unit.*

Sanjay: *This band 6 registered nurse did not demonstrate adequate knowledge in relation to the administration of medicines in the nursing home where he was employed. He failed to comply with the organisation's policy on medicines administration and left unattended medicines on a patient's locker, which resulted in a different patient swallowing the medicine.*

Christy: *Christy failed to check a patient's identity correctly, which resulted in the wrong patient being given medication, which led to an extended length of stay in hospital.*

According to the National Patient Safety Agency (NPSA, 2007b), most medications are administered safely and effectively, but errors can and do occur at all stages of the medication process. The NPSA goes on to discuss that as many as one in ten medicines prescribed, dispensed or administered may result in an error, and in some cases, such as those involving injectable medicines, the rate is much higher. Medication errors can occur during prescribing, checking, dispensing and administering. Medication errors can be distressing and potentially harmful to the patient and also stressful to the person involved in the administration of the medicine. Many healthcare professionals can be involved in medication management, but this chapter will focus on the implications for nurses. As you can see from the case study above, sometimes serious errors made while administering medicines can result not only in harm to the patient but also in registrants being suspended or removed from the professional regulatory body's register. This chapter will start by defining medication errors and discussing potential harms from medicine errors. We will then go on to look at why errors occur. We will focus on the administration of insulin as an example of good practice principles in relation to medicines administration, then go on to explore reporting and learning from incidents. We will conclude by offering tips for good practice, incorporating professional and legislative guidelines.

Medicines management covers a wide range of issues, which are outlined in much of the literature. We have suggested a selection of further reading at the end of the chapter to enhance your knowledge and understanding.

Activity 4.1   *Reflection*

- Consider how medication errors might occur. Write down and compare your list with suggestions we have made in the answers to activities at the end of the chapter.

We will begin to look at how medication errors may occur in more detail throughout the chapter.

What is a medication safety incident?

According to the National Patient Safety Agency (NPSA), many terms have been used to describe medication incidents and below is a summary of these terms.

- Medication errors

Medication errors are incidents in which there has been an error in the process of prescribing, dispensing, preparing, administering, monitoring or providing medicine advice, regardless of whether any harm occurred. This is a broad definition and most errors do not result in harm.

- Potential harms from medicines (near misses)

The incident may not have caused harm but did have the potential to cause harm. Near misses provide an insight into risk and areas where systems may be improved.

- Harm from medicines

Actual harm or adverse drug events can be categorised as preventable or non-preventable. For example, where a patient suffers harm from a medicine that was unforeseeable, this is categorised as an adverse drug event.

Errors in medicines administration

In Activity 4.1 you may have listed a combination of factors that may contribute to medication error. Some of these may be classified as system failures, whereas others may be caused by human error. We will be exploring these concepts in more detail in Chapter 7.

Common contributory factors leading to medicine errors are:

- incorrect prescribing;
- incorrect dispensing;
- failure to adhere to policy and procedures when managing and administering medicines;
- incorrect identification of patients;
- lack of knowledge in relation to the medicine (correct dose, interactions, side effects);
- incorrect dose/calculation error;
- wrong route of administration;
- failure to monitor patients for adverse reactions.

Errors in medicines administration occur in a variety of settings and relate to a wide range of medicinal products. The administration of insulin is one procedure where safety is a current area of focus. Therefore, we have chosen to focus on the administration and management of insulin in the next section of the chapter. Many of the principles and good practice that will be discussed in relation to the safe administration and management of insulin are transferable to other medicines.

Errors in medicines administration: application to practice and the administration of insulin

As you will be aware, insulin is a potent, life-saving medication that is an essential part of the daily regime for many people with diabetes. In 2010 it was estimated that there were 3,099,853 people in England with diabetes (APHO, 2010). It is worth noting that people or patients under the age of 18 who have diabetes and use insulin are not considered within the scope of this chapter as this area is so specialised.

In 2007 the NPSA published a report from the Patient Safety Observatory (PSO), *Safety in Doses: Medication safety incidents in the NHS* (NPSA, 2007c). In this report insulin was noted to be one of the medicines most commonly associated with incidents leading to severe harm or death. Insulin is frequently included in the list of top ten high-alert medicines worldwide.

If we explore the common contributing factors specifically to errors associated with insulin, the top three types of error are:

- wrong dose;
- omitted medicine;
- wrong insulin product.

Stage	Number	Percentage (%)
Administration	9,274	61
Prescribing	2,516	17
Dispensing and preparation	1,604	11
Monitoring of medicine use	771	5
Other	1,062	6
Total	15,227	100

Table 4.1: Stages of medication process where incidents involving insulin took place (Patient Safety First, 2010b)

The three categories highlighted accounted for 61 per cent of 15,227 incidents reported between November 2003 and August 2009 that involved insulin.

Case study

Agnes was a 94-year-old lady who was an insulin-dependent diabetic. She was almost totally blind as a result of her diabetes and required district nursing assistance with the administration of her insulin, twice a day. Agnes lived alone in a small bungalow and was relatively independent, managing her own housework and only relying on her son and daughter-in-law for grocery shopping.

On 18 September at 0830, Brenda, the district nurse, called by to give Agnes her injection of insulin. When Brenda arrived at the bungalow she realised that she did not have the appropriate insulin syringe required. She did, however, have an ordinary syringe. Brenda felt that she was competent to undertake the calculation required in order to administer the prescribed dose of insulin, taking into account the different size of syringe.

Agnes required 24 international units of insulin. Brenda administered what she considered to be 24 international units of insulin, documenting that the insulin had been given. Brenda left Agnes to start her breakfast.

At 1200 Agnes's son called with some fresh milk and bread. He found Agnes slumped in her chair and was unable to rouse her. He immediately called the emergency services; they arrived promptly but unfortunately it was too late to attempt to resuscitate Agnes.

The Coroner's inquest revealed that Agnes had suffered from severe hypoglycaemia resulting in a heart attack. It was found that Agnes had been administered ten times the prescribed dose of insulin (240 international units). The inquest ruled that Agnes had been unlawfully killed.

What we can see from this case study is that some mistakes can be fatal. Events like these are not everyday occurrences but we must acknowledge the fact that they can and do happen. The effects of harming a patient can be widespread. A fatal error or mistake that results in harming a patient can have devastating emotional and physical consequences for all those involved.

Activity 4.2   *Critical thinking*

- Think about a time when you have made a mistake. This could be forgetting about a dental appointment or arriving at the station only to find that the train has already left.
- Think about how this mistake made you feel emotionally.
- Did this mistake result in any physical consequences for yourself or another person?

As this activity is based on your own thoughts and feelings, there is no answer at the end of the chapter.

Incidents that have caused harm, or reports of death involving people or patients with diabetes, have been widely reported by the media. It is understandable that publicity of this nature potentially leads to a loss of confidence in the standard of care delivered, has negative effects on staff morale and decreases public confidence in the NHS.

Scenario

Imagine that you are a student nurse allocated to the practice area where the incident involving Agnes and Brenda took place (see case study). Take some time to think about the implications of the case study.

What might this mean:

- *for the family;*
- *for the individual nurse and the nursing profession;*
- *in relation to long-term impact for other diabetic people;*
- *for other patients, families, carers and nurses alike?*

The implications for the case study involving Agnes and Brenda are far reaching. You may well have considered each group individually, for example.

- **The family** – the traumatic loss of a loved one under circumstances they had no control over. They may feel cheated in some way and they may feel that they want to 'blame' someone and for that person to be punished for his or her inappropriate behaviour and/or actions.
- **The individual nurse** – she will have to live with the fact that she has made the fatal mistake for the rest of her life. The likelihood is that she would be unable to work as a registrant. The nurse may also face criminal charges and prosecution. Although sorry and remorseful, the nurse would never be able to console the family with such sentiments. The mistake could lead to physical consequences for the nurse such as depression.
- **The nursing profession** – the public's high regard for the profession is brought into question. Negative effects of adverse publicity can inhibit and undermine the nursing profession's growth.
- **The long-term impact** – those people, and to a large extent carers and families who know individuals living with diabetes, lose overall confidence in relation to their treatment plans. They want to be in control and manage their own medication wherever possible.

This is not an exhaustive list and you may well have considered other implications.

From reporting to learning

The value of reporting errors and mistakes was explored more comprehensively in Chapter 3, but essentially reporting is fundamental in preventing errors and mistakes from occurring again. When an error or mistake has been made that had the potential to, or did in fact cause harm, important information can often be provided. This information could well form the basis of a policy or procedure that may prevent a similar error from harming future patients.

In 2010 the NPSA, through reporting, recognised that errors in the administration of insulin were common. They also acknowledged that in certain cases they might be severe and cause death. Two common errors were identified.

- The inappropriate use of non-insulin (IV) syringes, which are marked in ml (millilitres) and not in insulin units (as in the case study above, where the wrong dose of insulin caused death).
- The use of abbreviations such as 'U' or 'IU' for units. When abbreviations are added to the intended dose, the dose may be misread, for example 10U could be read as 100. An example of this type of mistake is provided. The prescription is for Actrapid 4 units, but as you can see this could be misinterpreted as Actrapid 40.

ONCE ONLY

Date	Time	Drug (approved name)	Dose	Route	Prescriber's signature	Time given	Given by	Checked by	Pharm.
15.10.12	10.00	Actrapid	40	SC	J Smith				

Figure 4.1: An example of a drug kardex

Activity 4.3   *Evidence-based practice and research*

- Try to find out something about the policy or protocol for the administration of insulin in the hospital or community-based setting in which you are placed. You might also like to consider exploring policies and protocols within other practice areas in which you have worked, in order to get an overview of different approaches or interpretations. You might find that there is a 'standard' approach that is policy driven.
- Try to locate insulin syringes within your current practice area. You might want to carefully consider the difference between an insulin syringe and a non-insulin (IV) syringe.

As this activity is based on your own observation, there is no answer at the end of the chapter.

The NPSA clearly states that some of the errors have resulted from insufficient training in the use of insulin by healthcare professionals. In 2010 NHS Diabetes published *Safe and Effective Use of Insulin in Hospitalised Patients* and reinforced that the central reason for error is the lack of healthcare professional experience and knowledge of the use of insulin. They suggest that the number of incidents involving insulin can be greatly reduced by introducing and following a number of key principles, including the following.

- All healthcare professionals should receive regular education and training, with particular emphasis on patient safety. The potential for mistakes to occur should also be highlighted and how these mistakes have consequences for all those involved, particularly the patient.
- Protocols and checklists should be developed. (www.patientsafetyfirst.nhs.uk recommends using a care bundle in relation to high-risk medications: *Check the meds* – at the website, click 'Implementation', then 'One step to patient safety', then click 'Check the meds' on the list provided. You may want to revisit Chapter 2 at this point to remind yourself of the value of using bundles, protocols and checklists in your practice area. In essence, a bundle is an effort to design a standard approach. Your practice area may well have introduced a simple 'insulin prescription bundle'.)
- A second person should check all actions associated with the preparation and administration of insulin products.
- Communication should be improved between healthcare professionals and with diabetic patients.
- Electronic recording and prescribing should be in place.
- There should be discharge planning.

It is worth noting that the control of blood glucose is seen as a priority and is not secondary to the management of the initial cause for admission. For example, if someone who is insulin dependent is admitted to a secure unit for treatment of psychosis under the Mental Health Act 2007, a balanced approach must be considered to treat both the diabetes and the psychosis.

NHS Diabetes recognises that many patients who normally control their own diabetes find that, when they are admitted to hospital, they need to give up the control they have of managing their own diabetes to inexperienced nurses. This leads to anxiety and frustration for the patient, and an increased likelihood of an error, mistake or omission in relation to the overall management of their insulin-dependent diabetes.

Case study

Amit, aged 24, is admitted to ward 3 for arthroscopy and meniscectomy of his left knee. He was diagnosed with Type 1 diabetes at the age of 18, and although at first he struggled with his diagnosis he very quickly managed to adapt his lifestyle and routines. Amit was advised to attend the Dose Adjustment For Normal Eating (DAFNE) programme, which provided him with the skills necessary to estimate the carbohydrate in each meal and to inject the right dose of insulin. Amit found the programme extremely useful as it made him feel in control of his diabetes and lifestyle, rather than him changing his lifestyle to fit in with his diabetes.

During the admissions process, Steve, an experienced staff nurse, asked Amit questions in relation to his diabetes. Amit explained that he had been 'nil by mouth' from midnight in preparation for his operation and had therefore omitted his morning insulin. He also highlighted the fact that he liked to be in control of his diabetes. Steve asked Amit if he had brought his insulin into hospital, because if he had he would need to take

continued . . .

it from him. Amit said that he had brought his insulin pen with him and that he would prefer to administer his own medication. Steve claimed that it was not permitted for patients to administer their own medication and that his insulin would be given by the nursing staff. Steve asked Amit to hand over his insulin pen, which Amit did reluctantly.

Amit's surgery went well and without any difficulties. On return to the ward from the recovery area Steve told Amit that he could eat and drink. Amit asked if he could check his blood glucose level and that he would need some insulin before he had anything to eat. At that moment Steve was called away by the orthopaedic consultant, who wanted to undertake a ward round. Amit waited but Steve did not return. Amit felt frustrated and no longer in control of his own diabetes, his morning dose of insulin was omitted due to the fact he was 'nil by mouth', and now that he was able to eat he had no insulin to give himself. He tried to catch the attention of other staff on the ward but they were busy with patients who were either going to theatre or returning. Amit was unable to eat the sandwich that he was given because he had not received his insulin. A further dose of insulin had been omitted.

From this case study we can see how easy it is to omit medications. As nurses we can lose focus or become distracted; we are often placed in positions where we have to multitask, doing two or three things simultaneously. Steve was the senior staff nurse on duty, it was a busy theatre day and the orthopaedic consultant wanted to undertake a ward round. Steve would not have intentionally omitted Amit's insulin. Steve might have felt pressured and perhaps overwhelmed. Because he had to consider so many demands at one time he might have lost focus as to the importance of Amit receiving his insulin in a timely manner. This created a situation that put Amit at risk of harm. Amit was more than competent and it was safe for him to take control of his own medication.

Scenario

You might want to consider the outcome for Amit if he had been allowed to self-administer his insulin.

- *What might you need to consider at ward level if you allowed Amit to take control of the management of his diabetes?*
- *What could the consequences be for other insulin-dependent diabetic patients on the ward?*
- *What are the implications for staff on the ward?*

If Amit had been allowed to self-administer his insulin, he would have been able to eat and subsequently manage and control his blood glucose level. He had already experienced a period of time when he was unable to eat because of having to be 'nil by mouth' for his operation. Amit was competent and capable of self-administration; he had also attended DAFNE, which educates insulin-dependent diabetics to adjust their insulin in accordance with carbohydrate intake. Amit would not have experienced a sense of frustration and it would also have taken pressure off the busy nursing team by allowing Amit to manage his own diabetes.

For Amit to self-administer his insulin the ward would need to ensure that a robust policy or protocol was in place to allow this to happen. Key points for consideration might include the following.

- The safe and appropriate storage of insulin when it is not in use.
- The availability of appropriate equipment, such as insulin syringes and needles for injection, and subsequent safe disposal.
- Patients signing consent forms to indicate their willingness to self-manage their diabetes in hospital.
- A robust nursing assessment of patients to ensure competence in the management of their diabetes, including **sick day rules**, having a stable conscious level and reasonably stable insulin requirements, as well as the physical ability to self-monitor and/or inject. Circumstances may change during the inpatient stay and staff should be prepared to reassess the capability of the patient depending on the situation.
- The patient completing appropriate documentation when insulin has been self-administered.
- An appropriate policy that could be followed.
- Appropriate documentation and records being kept up to date and readily available to the patient and staff.
- The patient being assessed for competence and safe practice in relation to self-administration of insulin.
- All insulin products being stored appropriately and any equipment needed being available and, after use, disposed of safely.

This is not an exhaustive list and you may well have considered other implications.

Learning from these incidents

Through reporting, we have already established that insulin is one of the top ten high-alert medicines worldwide and the three most commonly associated errors. It seems that these errors are more likely to occur when we take control from the person or patient. To prevent situations like those highlighted in the case study from remaining commonplace in the practice area, we need to learn from mistakes and put mechanisms or processes in place to minimise the likelihood of them happening again.

We also need to consider our relationship or partnership with patients and if a patient controls and manages his or her own diabetes and is competent and safe to do so, it would be more appropriate for control to remain with the patient if admitted to a hospital setting.

The NPSA (2011b) issued a Patient Safety Alert, *The Adult Patient's Passport to Safer Use of Insulin*. The Director of Patient Safety said:

> *Medication incidents continue to be a leading cause of harm in healthcare. With insulin this can lead to serious harm or death. The Insulin Passport offers patients and healthcare professionals a simple tool to help reduce that risk.*

The main focus of the Patient Safety Alert is to give control to patients with diabetes, allowing them to take a more active role in their treatment and to avoid being given the wrong insulin.

The Patient Safety Alert also asks for systems to be in place enabling hospital inpatients to self-administer insulin. Obviously, not every inpatient will be competent or be able to self-administer insulin and this would form an important part of the nursing assessment. By allowing patients to take control it is believed that this should reduce the number of mistakes associated with incorrect timing of insulin administration with food. It may also reduce the harm caused by missed doses, such as when patients are 'nil by mouth'.

Insulin Passport and patient information booklet

By 31 August 2012 the NPSA hoped that all NHS organisations would have adopted and implemented some key principles in relation to safer use of insulin for adults. The vision is that the patient information booklet and the Insulin Passport will complement existing systems that might already be in place, ensuring key information is easily accessed across healthcare sectors about individual patients and their insulin requirements.

The key principles were that, by 31 August 2012, the following would be in place.

- Adult patients on insulin therapy would receive a patient information booklet and an Insulin Passport to help provide accurate identification of their current insulin products and provide essential information across healthcare sectors.
- Healthcare professionals and patients would be informed how the Insulin Passport-associated patient information can be used to improve safety.
- When prescriptions of insulin are prescribed, dispensed or administered, healthcare professionals would cross-reference available information to confirm the correct identity of insulin products.
- Systems would be in place to enable hospital inpatients to self-administer insulin where feasible and safe.

The Insulin Passport

The Insulin Passport is a single, double-sided sheet that folds up to credit-card size. It contains the necessary information for emergencies and safe use of insulin as patients transfer across healthcare providers. For example, when Amit was admitted to hospital he would be able to take with him his Insulin Passport. This would have provided vital information for Steve in relation to Amit's insulin therapy.

The patient information booklet

The patient information booklet explains the main purpose of the Insulin Passport. It also highlights the importance of keeping the Insulin Passport up to date. Key considerations for improving safety are clearly and simplistically discussed and include:

- the **correct storage** of insulin;
- the **right insulin** – check the name;
- the **right dose** – check the strength and how much insulin should be given;
- the **right time** – check the time for insulin administration;
- the **right way** – via syringe, pen or pump.

The patient information booklet emphasises that the Insulin Passport is to be used to 'help others do the right thing', but that patients have a responsibility to keep their Insulin Passports with them at all times and that they must be kept up to date.

Activity 4.4   *Evidence-based practice and research*

- Try to find out if your practice area is either aware of, or is using, the key principles of the Insulin Passport in relation to the safer use of insulin for adults. You might already have your answer if you completed Activity 4.3.
- Try to find out if hospital inpatients are able to self-administer insulin, and if so look at the 'systems' in place to allow this to happen. You might want to consider situations when it would not be feasible or safe for a hospital inpatient to self-administer insulin. You might find it useful to discuss some of your observations with your practice mentor.

As this activity is based on your own observation, there is no answer at the end of the chapter.

Case study

Daisy is an 88-year-old woman who was admitted to hospital from her care home after developing pneumonia, which required treatment with intravenous antibiotics. Daisy had been an insulin-dependent diabetic for many years and her diabetes was well controlled with twice-daily injections of Humalog Mix insulin. During her hospital stay the nursing staff managed Daisy's insulin injections and, now that Daisy was ready for discharge to the care home, she knew that the staff there would continue to manage her diabetes.

Katie, the Foundation Year 2 doctor, was asked to write a prescription for Daisy in preparation for her discharge. Katie was in the process of writing the prescription when she was called to attend a cardiac arrest. Katie had completed the prescription anyway and this was sent to the pharmacy so that all Daisy's medications could be prepared for her forthcoming transfer to the care home.

Daisy was transferred back to the care home the following morning and she settled very quickly into her familiar surroundings. Sandra, the nurse in charge, checked Daisy's blood sugar and gave her the prescribed amount of insulin. Shortly after Daisy had finished her breakfast she began to feel shaky and dizzy. She called for Sandra, who had the insight to check Daisy's blood sugar. Daisy's blood sugar level had dropped to 2.8mmol/l and Sandra realised that Daisy was suffering from hypoglycaemia. Sandra quickly asked Daisy to chew two glucose tablets, which would provide some carbohydrate necessary to raise Daisy's blood sugar level. Sandra was concerned as this type of episode was not normal for Daisy following administration of her insulin.

Once Daisy was feeling better and her blood sugar level was 4.2mmol/l, Sandra checked the insulin that she had given Daisy earlier that morning and realised that it was the wrong insulin product. Daisy had been prescribed Humalog (rapid) and not Humalog Mix. Sandra phoned Daisy's GP practice asking for an urgent new prescription for Humalog Mix.

Problems can arise at transfer of care from hospital to the community. This case study highlights the potential for the wrong insulin products to be prescribed. Different manufacturers can make similar insulin products and there is a risk that patients may be given the wrong insulin. There are many different types of insulin with names that look and sound like one another.

Activity 4.5   *Critical thinking*

- You might want to consider how different the outcome would have been for Daisy if an Insulin Passport were in use.

As this activity is based on your own critical thinking, there is no answer at the end of the chapter.

We have focused on insulin as the scenarios and case studies we used illustrate some of the key principles of safe practice. There are, of course, a number of reported incidents in which errors have occurred when medicine has been administered. We shall now explore other scenarios that commonly occur in healthcare settings.

Case study

Omar is a 3-year-old boy who was admitted to the children's ward at 1100 on a Sunday morning. He was fretful and feverish and he also had a rash on his body. On examination, the staff observed that the rash was **petechial** *in nature, which was suggestive of meningitis, and therefore a lumbar puncture was arranged and intravenous antibiotics were prescribed. The doctor prescribed intravenous penicillin but he put the decimal point in the wrong place. The prescription sheet was handwritten and the writing unclear as if he had written it in a rush. The nurse about to administer the medication realised this and queried it with the doctor. The doctor, realising his potentially dangerous mistake, corrected the prescription and averted a potentially serious error.*

The nurse averted a potential error because not only did she have knowledge of the correct dosage of this medicine, but she was also concerned about the legibility of the prescription. There are a number of reported incidences where the wrong dose of medicine was prescribed and sometimes it is simply that the decimal point was put in the wrong place or obscured by illegible handwriting. Electronic prescribing is now being introduced to many healthcare organisations, which may help to avoid errors in interpreting handwriting. However, what is important here is that the nurse recognised an anomaly with the prescribed dose and she also questioned it.

Case study

Ada, a 70-year-old former nurse, had been making an uneventful recovery from a total knee replacement when she was given intravenous Augmentin. Within one minute of administration she began to develop difficulty in breathing and marked angioedema of her face. Immediate action was taken but she developed respiratory distress and, despite repeated attempts to resuscitate her, she died. Ada was allergic to penicillin and this was recorded in her notes but had not been noticed by staff.

There are a number of issues contributing to patient safety here, the most obvious being failure to check the documentation to ascertain whether the patient had any known allergies. There are other locally agreed policies in place to identify patients with known allergies, such as wrist bands and alert labels, which are visible around the patient's environment.

Case study

Jane works in the community and, while visiting Edwin, who is a palliative care patient, she requests a change of analgesia from the GP whom she contacts on her mobile phone. The GP gives a verbal message over the phone to increase Edwin's existing analgesia.

A verbal order is not acceptable on its own. The NMC provides guidance and recommends that:

> *in exceptional circumstances, a medical practitioner may need to prescribe remotely for a previously unprescribed medicine, for example, in palliative care or remote rural areas the use of information technology (such as fax, text message or email) must confirm the prescription before it is administered. This should be followed up by a new prescription signed by the prescriber who sent the fax/email confirming the changes within normally a maximum of 24 hours (72 hours maximum [allowing for] bank holidays and weekends). The registrant is accountable for ensuring all relevant information has been communicated to the prescriber and s/he may refuse to accept a remote prescription if it compromises care to the patient. In this instance s/he should document accurately the communication that has taken place. Registrants should note that remote prescribing cannot be undertaken in a care home because they do not have access to a stock of medicines.*
> (NMC, 2010d, p29)

Activity 4.6 *Reflection*

- What policies and procedures exist in your own organisation to identify patients with known allergies?

As this activity relates to your own organisation, there is no answer at the end of the chapter.

Healthcare Trusts and organisations must incorporate standards and directives in their safety frameworks. Though there will be variations from one organisation to another, the key principles should remain the same.

NMC *Standards for Medicines Management*

The Nursing and Midwifery Council (2010d) has set out standards for management of medicines that cover a wide range of activities from prescribing to dispensing, administration, storage and disposal. You are advised to read this document and familiarise yourself with its contents. It is not enough to rely on your mentor in practice alone to tell you what the expected standards are. Make sure you have the most up-to-date version as the NMC revises its standards regularly, as they are reviewed and updated in line with legislation and practice (www.nmc-uk.org).

It is not within the scope of this chapter to cover all aspects of the document, but we will focus specifically on some standards in relation to checking and administering medicines.

Section 1: Method of supplying and/or administration of medicines (p18)

Standard 2: Checking

1. Registrants (1st and 2nd level) must check any direction to administer a medicinal product.
2. As a registrant you are accountable for your actions and omissions. In administering any medication, or assisting or overseeing any self-administration of medication, you must exercise your professional judgement and apply your knowledge and skill in the given situation. As a registrant, before you administer a medicinal product you must always check that the prescription or other direction to administer:
   2.1 is not for a substance to which the patient is known to be allergic or is otherwise unable to tolerate;
   2.2 is based, whenever possible, on the patient's informed consent and awareness of the purpose of the treatment;
   2.3 is clearly written, typed or computer-generated and indelible;
   2.4 specifies the substance to be administered, using its generic or brand name where appropriate and its stated form, together with the strength, dosage, timing, frequency of administration, start and finish dates, and route of administration;
   2.5 is signed and dated by the authorised prescriber;
   2.6 specifies, in the case of controlled drugs, the dosage and the number of dosage units or total course; and is signed and dated by the prescriber using relevant documentation as introduced, for example, patient drug record cards.
3. In addition, you must have:
   3.1 clearly identified the patient for whom the medication is intended;
   3.2 recorded the weight of the patient on the prescription sheet, if the patient is a child, or where the dosage of medication is related to the patient's weight or surface area (for example, in the case of cytotoxics) or where clinical condition dictates.

Section 4: Standards for practice of administration of medicines (pp23–4)

1. Having initially checked the direction to supply or administer that a medicinal product is appropriate for your patient or client (standard 2) you may then administer medication.

Standard 8: Administration

2. As a registrant, in exercising your professional accountability in the best interests of your patients:

2.1 you must be certain of the identity of the patient to whom the medicine is to be administered;

2.2 you must check that the patient is not allergic to the medicine before administering it;

2.3 you must know the therapeutic uses of the medicine to be administered, its normal dosage, side effects, precautions and contra-indications;

2.4 you must be aware of the patient's plan of care (care plan or pathway);

2.5 you must check that the prescription or the label on the medicine dispensed is clearly written and unambiguous;

2.6 you must check the expiry date (where it exists) of the medicine to be administered;

2.7 you must have considered the dosage, weight where appropriate, method of administration, route and timing;

2.8 you must administer or withhold in the context of the patient's condition (for example, Digoxin is not usually given if a patient's pulse is below 60 beats per minute) and co-existing therapies, for example, physiotherapy;

2.9 you must contact the prescriber or any other authorised prescriber without delay where contra-indications to the prescribed medicine are discovered, where the patient develops a reaction to the medicine or where assessment of the patient indicates that the medicine is no longer suitable (see standard 25);

2.10 you must make a clear, accurate and immediate record of all medicine administered, intentionally withheld or refused by the patient, ensuring that the signature is clear and legible; it is also your responsibility to ensure that a record is made when delegating the task of administering medicine.

How can I ensure that I maintain safety when administering medicines and medicine products?

Medicines management is a wide subject area and it is not within the scope of this book to cover all aspects. We recommend that you read O'Brien et al. (2011) *Introduction to Medicines Management in Nursing,* which aims to specifically support nursing students on nursing undergraduate programmes in relation to medicines management.

In order to practise medicines management safely, it is imperative that you develop the necessary knowledge and skills to underpin your practice. These are illustrated in Figure 4.2.

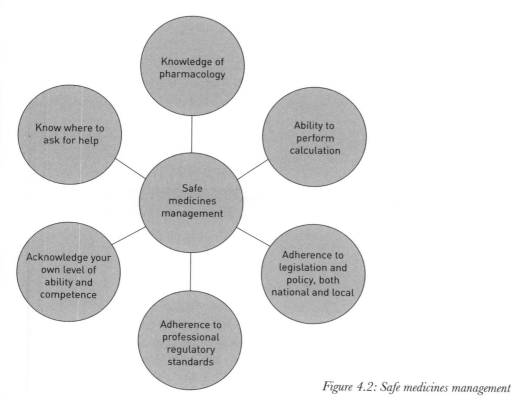

Figure 4.2: Safe medicines management

Knowledge and skills

- Knowledge of pharmacology

As a registered nurse or midwife, you should have sufficient knowledge about any medicine product you administer in order to do so safely and effectively. This includes: correct dose, route of administration and method of administration, as well as potential adverse reactions, and potential or known interactions.

- Practice according to legislation and policy

You must be aware of policies and guidelines set by your employer. Do not rely on your colleagues to tell you what the policy states – read it yourself!

- Professional standards

Practise within the requirements of regulatory standards such as those set by the NMC.

- Perform calculations safely and accurately

It is imperative that nurses are able to perform calculations. There are a number of tools and training packages available to help you with your numeracy skills if required. Your own university or placement provider will be able to advise you on this.

- Know where to seek advice

There are a number of people who can advise you if you are unsure about administering a medicine. If in doubt – ASK! Many hospitals, clinics and pharmacies have information pharmacists who can help you if you are unsure about a dose, route of administration and so on.

- Acknowledge your own level of competence and knowledge

Be self-aware. If you lack knowledge in an area of practice, acknowledge it and seek support. As a student there are a number of people who can support you and give advice, including mentors and educators in practice, lecturers and study skills services in your university. Develop skills to remain focused when administering medicines as distractions can interfere with concentration and accuracy.

Activity 4.8   *Evidence-based practice and research*

In relation to you as a student administering medicines, what do the following organisational policies state:

- the Nursing and Midwifery Council;
- your university;
- your placement provider?

As this activity is based on your individual organisation, there is no answer at the end of the chapter.

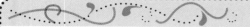

Chapter summary

This chapter has explored issues associated with the safe administration of medicines. We have provided a brief introduction to safe medicines administration and this chapter should be read in conjunction with the standards and policies set out by your professional regulatory body and employing organisation. We have given you some ideas on which you can build your own knowledge base in relation to safe practice, specifically the skills you require to practise safely.

Activities: brief outline answers

Activity 4.1: Reflection (page 63)

Errors may occur due to the following (the list is not exhaustive):

- incorrect prescribing;
- wrong patient;
- incorrect medicine;
- incorrect dose calculation;
- failure to check allergies;
- wrong route of administration;
- incorrect setting of medical device to administer medicine;
- incorrect documentation and recording.

Further reading

Nursing and Midwifery Council (NMC) (2010) *Standards for Medicines Management*. NMC: London. Available at www.nmc-uk.org/Documents/NMC-Publications/NMC-Standards-for-medicines-management. pdf.

The NMC provide standards that all nursing students and registrants must abide by. You can access the most updated version by visiting the NMC website. Copies are available in hard format and you can also download.

O'Brien, M, Spires, A and Andrews, K (2011) *Introduction to Medicines Management in Nursing*. Exeter: Learning Matters.

This is a comprehensive and straightforward text that can help you understand your role and responsibilities in relation to medicines administration.

Useful websites

www.bnf.org

This website offers the reader access to information about medicines and is comprehensive. At this time, user registration is required at no charge.

www.diabetes.nhs.uk/safety

This website provides an essential link between diabetes strategy and frontline service improvements for patients. The overall aim is to champion good-quality diabetes care. There is a range of resources, which will support your learning in relation to diabetes care and information about safety work programmes. This is a very comprehensive website that provides free online access for completing an e-learning module on 'Safe Use of Insulin'. You can also access information about the Insulin Passport and the patient information booklet.

www.nrls.npsa.nhs.uk/resources/?EntryId45=130397

This link will take you directly to the NHS safety alert, which provides key information in relation to the Insulin Passport. The principles outlined in the Insulin Passport should be available across all healthcare sectors by the time of writing.

www.patientsafetyfirst.nhs.uk

This is a very comprehensive website that has evolved over time to become a 'hub' for a number of patient safety improvement programmes and resources, for example evaluation reports in relation to patient safety initiatives.

Chapter 5
Raising concerns: safeguarding the vulnerable

> ### NMC Standards for Pre-registration Nursing Education
>
> This chapter will address the following competencies:
>
> **Domain 1: Professional values**
>
> 1. All nurses must practise with confidence according to *The Code: Standards of conduct, performance and ethics for nurses and midwives* (NMC, 2008), and within other recognised ethical and legal frameworks. They must be able to recognise and address ethical challenges relating to people's choices and decision making about their care, and act within the law to help them and their families and carers find acceptable solutions.
>
> 1.1 Adult nurses must understand and apply current legislation to all service users, paying special attention to the protection of vulnerable people, including those with complex needs arising from ageing, cognitive impairment, long-term conditions and those approaching the end of life.
>
> 2. All nurses must practise in a holistic, non-judgemental, caring and sensitive manner that avoids assumptions, supports social inclusion; recognises and respects individual choice; and acknowledges diversity. Where necessary, they must challenge inequality, discrimination and exclusion from access to care.
>
> 4. All nurses must work in partnership with service users, carers, families, groups, communities and organisations. They must manage risk, and promote health and well-being while aiming to empower choices that promote self-care and safety.
>
> 6. All nurses must understand the roles and responsibilities of other health and social care professionals, and seek to work with them collaboratively for the benefit of all who need care.
>
> **Domain 2: Communication and interpersonal skills**
>
> 2. All nurses must use a range of communication skills and technologies to support person-centred care and enhance quality and safety. They must ensure people receive all the information they need in a language and manner that allows them to make informed choices and share decision making. They must recognise when language interpretation or other communication support is needed and know how to obtain it.
>
> 4. All nurses must recognise when people are anxious or in distress and respond effectively, using therapeutic principles, to promote their well-being, manage personal safety and

continued . . .

resolve conflict. They must use effective communication strategies and negotiation techniques to achieve best outcomes, respecting the dignity and human rights of all concerned. They must know when to consult a third party and how to make referrals for advocacy, mediation and arbitration.

8. All nurses must respect individual rights to confidentiality and keep information secure and confidential in accordance with the law and relevant ethical and regulatory frameworks, taking account of local protocols. They must also actively share personal information with others when the interests of safety and protection override the need for confidentiality.

Domain 3: Nursing practice and decision making

7. All nurses must be able to recognise and interpret signs of normal and deteriorating mental and physical health and respond promptly to maintain or improve the health and comfort of the service user, acting to keep them and others safe.

Domain 4: Leadership, management and team working

7. All nurses must work effectively across professional and agency boundaries, actively involving and respecting others' contributions to integrated person-centred care. They must know when and how to communicate with and refer to other professionals and agencies in order to respect the choices of service users and others, promoting shared decision making, to deliver positive outcomes and to coordinate smooth, effective transition within and between services and agencies.

NMC Essential Skills Clusters

This chapter will address the following ESCs:

Cluster: Care, compassion and communication

7. People can trust the newly registered graduate nurse to protect and keep as confidential all information relating to them.

By the first progression point:

2. Protects and treats information as confidential except where sharing information is required for the purposes of safeguarding and public protection.

By entry to the register:

5. Acts professionally and autonomously in situations where there may be limits to confidentiality, for example, public interest and protection from harm.

6. Recognises the significance of information and acts in relation to who does or does not need to know.

7. Acts appropriately in sharing information to enable and enhance care (carers, MDT and across agency boundaries).

9. Acts within the law when confidential information has to be shared with others.

continued . . .

8. People can trust the newly registered graduate nurse to gain their consent based on sound understanding and informed choice prior to any intervention and that their rights in decision making and consent will be respected and upheld.

By the first progression point:

1. Seeks consent prior to sharing confidential information outside the professional care team, subject to agreed safeguarding and protection procedures.

By entry to the register:

7. Demonstrates respect for the autonomy and rights of people to withhold consent in relation to treatment within legal frameworks and in relation to people's safety.

Chapter aims

After reading this chapter, you will be able to:

- appreciate what is meant by the term safeguarding;
- understand why some people are vulnerable in the healthcare arena;
- glean an insight into how concerns can be raised in clinical practice if you are worried about a patient or client.

Introduction

Safeguarding adults: if you don't do something, who will?
(NMC, 2010e)

Scenario

Imagine you are visiting Mr Jones with the district nurse. Mr Jones is a 54-year-old man with a learning disability who lives with his sister and her husband plus their three grown-up children in a large five-bedroom house. He required dressings to a leg ulcer. His main carer is Anne, his sister, a rather intimidating woman in her sixties. Mr Jones is a quiet man who always smiles and is grateful for everything that is done for him. After you have finished his dressing, the district nurse is having a friendly chat with Mr Jones's brother-in-law. Anne comes out of the kitchen and walks towards Mr Jones. You notice him flinch and mutter something like 'Don't hurt me!', but you can't be sure. Anne laughs and goes up to him to make a fuss of him and give him a cup of tea and a biscuit. Mr Jones quietly says 'Thank you'. When you leave the house with the district nurse you ponder over whether you should mention it to her. However, the district nurse comments on what a lovely family they are and how caring Anne is towards her brother. You decide not to mention anything about the incident, thinking you had probably read more into it than existed.

continued . . .

- *How would you feel when you found out the next day that Mr Jones had been admitted to Accident and Emergency (A&E) with a head injury and black eye, which was suspected to be non-accidental?*
- *Do you think you may regret not mentioning what you had witnessed to the district nurse?*

This chapter has started with the above scenario to make you think about when it is appropriate to raise your concerns with other healthcare professionals. Sometimes, we can jump to conclusions without establishing any of the facts, and at other times we may overreact to situations and circumstances. This may prevent us from speaking up in subsequent situations. However, if you don't speak up, serious situations may go unnoticed and the consequences may be severe. The publication *Death by Indifference: 74 deaths and counting* (Mencap, 2012) confirms this. In the previous chapters we have discussed the safety of patients, focusing on error and mistakes. However, another aspect of safety that is increasingly becoming an area of concern in healthcare is that of safeguarding, and it is worth offering a chapter on this subject. We will start by looking at who might be vulnerable. The safeguarding of children has long been recognised as an area of priority in health and social care, and it is not within the scope of this chapter to explore the safeguarding of children in any detail. However, reference will be made to case studies involving children as some of the principles of good practice are transferable. It can be argued, however, that the safeguarding of adults in the health and social care system has, until recently, been rather implicit as opposed to explicit. So, with this in mind, we will explore what is meant by safeguarding and discuss some of the things that people need safeguarding from. We will look at types of abuse and explore who may inflict this abuse on the vulnerable and in particular the elderly. Some potential safeguarding situations are not always obvious, so finally we will look at strategies to help you identify when situations are of concern and how to raise your concerns to the most appropriate people.

A need for good safeguarding practice

A more detailed account of the issues of safeguarding can be found in Northway and Jenkins (2013).

It is acknowledged that all persons have the right to live their lives free from violence and abuse. This right is underpinned by the duty on public agencies under the law, including the Human Rights Act 1998, to intervene proportionately to protect the rights of citizens. These rights include Article 2: 'the right to life', Article 3: 'freedom from torture' (including humiliating and degrading treatment) and Article 8: 'the right to private and family life' (one that sustains the individual). People in our society need to feel safe and free from harm. They also expect to have support with a range of activities when they are unable to carry them out independently. This may vary from full-time care if a patient is affected by physical or mental illness or temporary care while he or she is incapacitated. The level of nursing care required will vary from person to person and is often delivered alongside other agencies. People need to be protected from harm by those caring for them and the last thing they need is to be abused by those charged with caring for them. Sadly, you will be aware that this does happen to some individuals. The report *No Secrets*, published by the Department of Health (2000b), gave local social services authorities lead responsibility for coordinating local multi-agency systems, policies and procedures to protect vulnerable adults from abuse. In October 2008 the Department of Health carried out a large national consultation on safeguarding adults from abuse and harm with the aim of establishing how far the *No Secrets* guidance had progressed and how it could be improved. One of the key findings was the absence of adult safeguarding systems within the NHS to ensure that healthcare incidents that raise safeguarding concerns are considered in the wider safeguarding arena.

Who commits abuse?

Safeguarding of the vulnerable adult or child can encompass a wide range of scenarios. Often it is the family member or carer who is the abuser, but more recently there have been reported cases involving healthcare workers as the perpetrators and, in some instances, what can be described as institutional abuse.

Safeguarding an individual from harm or abuse can relate to:

- physical abuse;
- sexual abuse;
- psychological abuse;
- financial abuse;
- neglect or acts of omission.

Activity 5.1   *Critical thinking*

- What kinds of adults or children do you think may be 'vulnerable' and require protection and why?
- What sorts of 'protection' might they require?

An outline answer is provided at the end of the chapter.

All of us are vulnerable at some time in our lives: vulnerable to harm, abuse or neglect. The most obvious age groups susceptible to vulnerability are the very young and the aged. Other people in society are also vulnerable, perhaps as a result of illness or disability. At the present time, there have been a number of media reports that have highlighted cases where vulnerable adults have been abused while in the care of health or social care organisations.

Activity 5.2 — *Critical thinking*

- With a peer, make a list of some of the high-profile safeguarding cases that have been reported in the media recently.
- Select one particular case study and see what you can find out about it. You might search news archives, journal articles and the internet. Be aware that the details of some of the cases you read about will be distressing.

As this activity is based on your own observation, there is no answer at the end of the chapter.

In 2012, six out of eleven care workers who admitted a total of 38 charges of neglect or abuse of patients at a private care home, Winterbourne View, were jailed. The hospital looked after vulnerable adults, many of whom had learning disabilities and some of whom displayed challenging behaviour. The systematic abuse of patients was uncovered by the BBC. Staff were found guilty of treatment that was described as cruel, callous and degrading. What is most disturbing about this case study is that the relatives of these victims entrusted their loved ones to the care of those employed to look after them. They were badly let down by those individuals and the system. The report can be accessed at www.bbc.co.uk/news/uk-england-bristol-20092894.

In contrast, the case of Peter Connelly, known as 'Baby P', and the subsequent dismissal of the Director of Haringey Council's Children's Services fundamentally changed the way in which children are protected from not only the wider public but also from those entrusted to care for them.

Case study

On 3 August 2007, Peter Connelly was found dead in his cot 48 hours after a doctor failed to spot the child's severe injuries, including a broken spine. The toddler was on the council's child protection register throughout eight months of abuse in which he suffered in excess of 50 injuries. There had been a number of agencies assigned to work with this family but none of them managed to prevent the progressive abuse that would eventually lead to his death. Ironically, Haringey Council had previously found itself at the centre of a public outcry over the murder of Victoria Climbié by her aunt and her aunt's boyfriend.

Of course the above cases received much media attention and fuelled public outcry. A number of reports, guidelines and publications followed.

Activity 5.3   *Reflection*

- Imagine you had been involved in the care of a child in similar circumstances to the above. How do you think you would feel as events unfolded?
- There were a number of agencies involved in the care of this family yet his death was not prevented. Do you think you have the necessary skills to speak out if you had suspected abuse was taking place?

As this activity is based on your own experience and feelings, there is no answer at the end of the chapter.

If you are a student nurse, you will be undertaking education and training in a particular field of nursing. You may feel that, as an adult nurse, it is unlikely that you will ever be involved in the care of a child. If you are in the field of children's nursing, you may feel that your involvement with vulnerable adults will be unlikely. However, whatever the field of nursing you are working in, you will be involved in the care of individuals and their families or carers. It is therefore important that you think holistically towards the family group, as the problems experienced by your individual patients or clients will undoubtedly have some sort of residual effect upon their families or carers. Safeguarding is every healthcare professional's concern. How, then, can it be approached?

Raising concerns

The Nursing and Midwifery Council (NMC) reminds us that it exists to safeguard the health and well-being of the public. This is achieved by maintaining a register of nurses, midwives and specialist community public health nurses. This will be discussed in more detail in the following chapter. The NMC has published guidance for its members so that they are aware of how they can raise and escalate concerns appropriately.

Case study

Daniel is a second-year student nurse on placement in a hospital that specialises in care for the elderly. His mentor is Helen, a band 6 staff nurse. Helen has been working at the hospital for over ten years and she is a good friend of the ward manager, Deb. Helen works a lot of nightshifts because she has a family and she prefers to work nights as the shifts suit her family routine. Daniel does not mind working night shifts as it allows him to experience the different needs of patients over the 24-hour period and, because many of the patients are dependent, the night shift is busy and there are plenty of opportunities to learn. Helen is a confident woman and she often takes charge of the shift. Some of the staff have commented that they find her bossy, but few of them challenge her as on the whole she is well respected and comes across as a bubbly, friendly lady who enjoys mentoring students. On his second week of night shift, Daniel is becoming increasingly concerned. Many of the patients are assessed as being at high risk of developing pressure ulcers. The ward manager is vigilant in

continued . . .

her approach to promoting tissue viability in her clinical area and all patients undergo a thorough and regular assessment of risk during their stay. The ward is also well equipped with pressure-relieving resources and all staff undertake regular training and updates to use the equipment. Many of the patients require two-hourly positional changes in their plan of care and this is documented in the care plan. Daniel is aware that two patients in particular, both of whom have dementia, require two-hourly positional changes. However, for three nights running, Helen has failed to change the position of the patients for six–seven hours. Daniel asked one of the healthcare assistants to help him move one patient, but she refused saying that the patients need their rest and they will come to no harm. He asks Helen again if she will help him move the patient and she responds by saying that she does not believe it is in the patient's best interests to disturb her sleep. She needs her rest and it is ridiculous to disturb the woman when she is so comfortable. She goes on to assert that in all her years of nursing she has never come across a patient who has developed a pressure ulcer when they have been turned less frequently on night shift, and that sometimes nurses need to 'use their common sense' instead of following what others demand all the time. He does note, however, that the record documenting positional change has been ticked and signed for at the end of the bed. When the patient was eventually moved, Daniel observed that her sacrum and heels appeared very red. When he commented on this to Helen, she replied that it was inevitable because the patient is a frail, elderly woman and her metabolism is sluggish and that he has no cause for concern because her nutritional status is good and she is not incontinent.

Activity 5.4 *Critical thiking*

- Imagine you are in Daniel's position. What sorts of issues arise in this case study?
- What options are open to Daniel to deal with this situation?
- Helen is an experienced nurse and well respected. She is also good friends with Deb, the ward manager. Could this have any significance?

We will explore the points raised in this activity further below.

This case study raises a number of issues, not the least of which is a failure to carry out care as directed in the plan of care for this patient. All care must be underpinned by a body of evidence and, of course, all nurses must use their skills of clinical decision making and professional judgement when deviating from the plan of care. However, in your opinion, do you think Helen has provided a sound rationale for her decision not to alter the patient's position? There is also the issue of falsifying documentation to suggest that frequent positional changes had been made. If the patient did, in fact, develop a pressure ulcer, this could escalate into a complaint and even litigation. The patient has dementia and therefore this adds to her vulnerability.

As a registrant you have a professional duty to report any concerns from your workplace that put the safety of the people in your care or the public at risk. The principles in the NMC guidance also apply to students and are underpinned by the document, *Guidance on Professional Conduct for Nursing and Midwifery Students* (NMC, 2010c).

It is likely that Daniel may feel uncomfortable in this situation and he may not find it easy to raise his concerns. The process may also seem quite daunting. Daniel could approach another member of staff on the ward and raise his concerns. Some students are allocated co-mentors so this might be a good starting point. Daniel may feel able to approach Deb, the ward manager. Deb might be a good friend of Helen but she is also her manager and a registrant, so she is bound by the requirements of the NMC and also her contract of employment. Daniel could also seek advice from his university tutor or lecturer. It is likely that his university faculty will have policy guidance for raising concerns. The placement area will also have a policy on raising and escalating concerns. Remember that raising a concern is different from making a complaint. Speaking up on behalf of people in your care is part of your role as a nurse. Doing nothing and perpetuating bad practice is not acceptable.

It is worthy of note that many safeguarding policies and guidelines refer to the development of decubitus (pressure) ulcers as an indicator of neglect. It is well known that certain individuals are at a higher risk of developing them because their susceptibility is increased. This could be as a result of poor nutritional status, certain diseases or poor health status in general. Nurses often complain of staff shortages preventing them from moving patients as frequently as they should. Could this, then, be seen as neglect? It is difficult to argue, but unless there is evidence to demonstrate that all necessary assessment, intervention and resources were put in place, which should of course be documented, the development of a pressure ulcer may well be viewed as a safeguarding issue.

Activity 5.5   *Reflection*

- See if you can access your university policy on raising concerns – sometimes known as 'whistleblowing'.
- Also take a look to see what your placement policy says on raising concerns.

Although this activity is based on your own placement, some suggestions can be found at the end of the chapter.

If you are raising a concern, you are worried generally about an issue, wrongdoing or risk that affects others. You are acting as a witness to what you have observed or to risks that have been reported to you. You are concerned that what you have observed could have an adverse effect on others and you are taking steps to draw attention to the issues. Making a complaint is different and, in these circumstances, you should follow the appropriate organisational policy. Chapter 6 will offer further discussion on professional accountability.

If you do need to raise a concern but you are unsure how to or cannot find the policy, the NMC (2010b) provides guidance on raising and escalating concerns. This can be accessed on the NMC website. You could also discuss your concern with one of the following:

- mentor or placement supervisor;
- lead nurse/clinical matron;
- personal tutor or lecturer;
- supervisor of midwives (if you are a midwifery student or midwife);

- line manager;
- consultant.

It is advisable to raise your concern with the individual involved but this is not always ideal or possible. You may then wish to discuss your concern with your line manager. Your concern may relate to the overall standard of care rather than the care of an individual patient and, in this instance, it is advisable to raise your concern with a senior member of staff, preferably a registrant who is concerned with professional standards. Your trade union or professional body can also offer support and advice during this process. It is advisable to put your concern in writing and ensure you keep a concise record.

Sometimes it can be information that is given to us by a relative or carer that escalates our concern about a patient or family member.

Case study

Sue is a child branch staff nurse and she has been caring for Natalie, a 7-year-old girl with a heart condition that required surgery. Natalie's mother, Jane, is staying with her in the side cubicle. Jane has another 15-year-old daughter at home with autism who is being looked after by her husband. Jane has built up a good relationship with Sue and often chats to her. One morning Jane appeared rather low in mood and Sue enquired what was wrong. Jane asked Sue not to tell anyone what she was about to say, but she had been finding it increasingly difficult to look after her elder daughter who had challenging behaviour. Now that she was a teenager, her behaviour had become worse and Jane confessed to wanting to beat her and had in fact kicked her on two occasions.

This is a complex situation. Jane had asked Sue to keep what she had told her to herself. The NMC *Code* (2008) states that people in your care have the right to confidentiality and the right to expect that the information they have given to a nurse or midwife is only used for the purpose for which it was given. Information should only be disclosed to a third party with consent. However, disclosures without consent can be justified if you feel that someone may be at risk of harm. These decisions are complex and each case must be viewed individually. In this situation, Sue could persuade Jane that she is concerned for both of them and feels that Jane may benefit from help, therefore seeking Jane's permission to disclose the information to another health or social care professional. Sue could also explain that she has a duty to safeguard and is obliged to disclose the information.

In complex situations such as this, you should seek advice from someone, preferably a senior member of staff who ideally is an NMC registrant. You should also be familiar with your Trust policy.

Safeguarding the elderly

The law does not necessarily distinguish between older and younger adults, but it is worth including a separate section here because in many developing countries people are living longer. We should surely celebrate being an ageing society, but there are also concerns that ageing is associated with a diminishing decline in functional capacity and general health, leading to an increase in utilisation of health and social care resources. Ageing is therefore often seen as a process of systematic stereotyping of, and discrimination against, old people (Wheeler, 2012). Arguably, chronological age is used as a systematic way of denying resources to people. Perhaps this then makes this group of patients potentially vulnerable, particularly if they lack mental capacity, are physically frail and have no means of advocacy. There is evidence that looking after the elderly is seen as a less attractive speciality for some nurses (Wheeler, 2012), yet many of the patients we look after are elderly. There have been many policies and frameworks developed to protect the elderly, but it is apparent that this group remains vulnerable to poor care and abuse in our society.

Case study

Joe is 79. He lives alone in a bungalow. He has a grown-up son and daughter who are both married with children. His daughter lives 170 miles away but his son lives fairly near to Joe. Joe recently suffered a stroke but after a period of rehabilitation he has returned to his own home. He is managing quite well. He can walk a short distance with the aid of a frame. He does need assistance with bathing. The community nursing team visit daily and he also has a home help. His daughter and son visit regularly and his son has taken over managing his affairs and finances. He also does his shopping for him. Beryl, the community staff nurse, has noticed that in recent weeks Joe has become withdrawn. He is not looking after himself, is forgetting to shave and he seems emaciated. She asks him about his food intake and he says that he is very hungry and that he is OK and not to fuss. When she looks in the fridge, it is almost empty. She observes that the bungalow feels cold and Joe has an extra cardigan on. She asks him why he has not turned the heating up and he says it is because it costs so much. She asks whether his son is still managing to do his shopping and pop in. Joe replies 'oh ay, when he's not spending it on himself' and changes the subject. She decides to keep an extra eye on him. Next day when Beryl visits, as she approaches the house she notices a car parked outside belonging to Joe's son. As she reaches the door she hears male voices shouting. She knocks briskly and enters the house. Joe appears withdrawn and afraid and his son appears angry as if they have just rowed. There is tension in the air and they both become quiet in Beryl's presence. Beryl enquires how everything is and engages Joe and his son in a benign conversation that clears the air. Beryl raises her concerns with Joe's son regarding his poor eating. He asks her into the kitchen to view the fridge. When they get to the kitchen his voice becomes weak and he makes disparaging remarks about Joe, saying she has no idea what he was like when he and his sister were younger. He was a bully, he would beat them and he abused his mother. He said that he felt obliged to look after him as he lived nearby, but that as far as he was concerned 'my father has had this coming to him for a long time!'

Abuse of the elderly can take many shapes and forms. What is happening in this case study and how far can Beryl take it? Is Joe's son behaving inappropriately towards his father? Is Joe vulnerable and is he at risk? Is this a family affair and one that Beryl should remain impartial about? It is clear that Beryl has a duty of care to Joe and she has to remain impartial and objective about the information she has been given. Does she now have a duty of care to Joe's son, who is clearly harbouring a lifelong secret and potential grudge. Does he need support? There are lots of questions here and there are a number of approaches Beryl can take, but as an experienced practitioner she will have to use her professional judgement in terms of how she will approach this. She may feel the need to pass this on to senior colleagues and meanwhile ensure that additional support is provided for Joe and offered to his son. Situations like this can be sensitive and each case must be addressed by taking into account a variety of factors. Beryl does have a duty of care to Joe and she must respond appropriately. What if this information was given to her in confidence? The NMC's *Code of Professional Conduct* (2002) requires that, as registrants, we must protect confidential information. Section 5.2 states:

> *You should seek patients' and clients' wishes regarding the sharing of information with their family and others. When a patient or client is considered incapable of giving permission, you should consult relevant colleagues.*
>
> (p7)

Section 5.3 states:

> *If you are required to disclose information outside the team that will have personal consequences for patients and clients, you must obtain their consent. If the patient or client withholds consent, or if consent cannot be obtained for whatever reason, disclosures may be made only where:*
>
> * *they can be justified in the public interest (usually where disclosure is essential to protect the patient or client or someone else from the risk of significant harm);*
> * *they are required by law or by order of a court.*
>
> (p7)

In complex situations like the one above, it is wise to seek advice from other professionals in conjunction with exercising your own professional decision making.

When does a situation become a concern?

Often nurses do not speak out because they are not sure if they should raise a concern or not. What may seem an issue to one person may be deemed acceptable to another.

Activity 5.6   *Critical thinking and decision making*

Consider the following scenarios and decide which, if any, you would action and raise a concern about.

- You are mentor to a student nurse who is late for duty one morning. She confides to you that her husband had hit her with the TV remote control and she needed to attend A&E to have a scalp wound glued. You know she has two young children.
- A patient with a mental health problem tells you that he wants to physically harm his wife because she has been physically abusing him for years.
- A registered nurse has been withdrawing medication from a patient on your ward because she thinks he should not be taking it and the doctor should not have prescribed the particular medicine.
- You observe the ward manager taking a patient's temperature without using a protective cover for the probe and she does not wash her hands between patients.
- A patient under the influence of alcohol strikes your colleague over the head and he instinctively hits him back.
- A nurse who is going through a messy divorce shouts and swears at a patient who has been rude to her.
- On the shift you have just worked, four patients were left for over an hour in soiled linen because a staff nurse and healthcare assistant had been sent home sick leaving the ward short staffed.

Because you are asked here to use your own decision making and professional judgement, there are no answers at the end of the chapter.

The scenarios should illustrate the complexities associated with deciding whether to report or not. There will inevitably be many factors you would need to take into consideration in each situation and this would shape your judgement. There are recognised hierarchies of abuse (Northway and Jenkins, 2013). At the top are physical and sexual abuses, probably because they are always viewed as serious and distressing. Psychological and financial abuses are often seen as less severe. Self-neglect is often viewed as victim blaming. If an elderly patient with capacity refuses care and treatment, this is their choice and it is difficult to implement safeguarding policies because there is no third party involved. Many people undertaking the activity above would feel compelled to report most of the situations, but there are some complex scenarios that may well evoke differences of opinion.

What is important is that as a student you seek advice and support. If you are a registrant and require advice in any given situation, remember that there are policies, guidelines and senior personnel who can support you in your decision making.

The law in relation to safeguarding

There is no one safeguarding law in existence. Rather, safeguarding adults is provided by a combination of acts and legislation. However, below are some examples of the legislative framework that drives safeguarding:

- Mental Health Act 1983 (amended 2007);
- Human Rights Act 1998;
- Domestic Violence Crimes and Victims Act 2004;
- Mental Capacity Act 2005;
- Health & Social Care Act 2008;
- Equality Act 2010;
- Social Care Bill 2011;
- Deprivation of Liberty Safeguards.

This is by no means an exhaustive list. Further information can be found in Northway and Jenkins (2013).

Although individuals and organisations may be aware of the policies and legislation that exist to safeguard vulnerable adults, barriers to implementation can and do exist. Often this is due to a lack of training and understanding, although safeguarding vulnerable adults is currently high on the agenda in NMC educational standards.

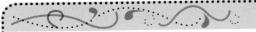

Chapter summary

This chapter has introduced you to the concept of safeguarding adults. Safeguarding is a complex area in healthcare and you are advised to engage in deeper reading around the subject and become familiar with policy and guidelines associated with protecting vulnerable adults. Safeguarding children is also a very complex area of practice and you are advised to familiarise yourself with local policy and procedures. What is clear is that, as healthcare professionals, we all have a responsibility to safeguard individuals with whom we come into contact through our professional roles. We must think beyond the patients or clients and consider the impact their illness or situation may have on their families or carers.

Activities: brief outline answers

Activity 5.1: Critical thinking (page 85)

You may have considered the following individuals to be vulnerable:

- adults who lack capacity;
- the elderly;
- people who are debilitated or incapacitated by illness or injury;
- children who are dependent on adults or under the age of 16;
- children in care;

- adults with learning disabilities;
- people with mental health problems;
- families and relatives of those who are incapacitated by illness or injury;
- adults who are financially or socially affected by illness or injury.

The vulnerable may require protection from:

- family members or carers;
- professionals or carers whose practice is substandard;
- other children;
- other adults.

Activity 5.5: Reflection (page 89)

Most university and Trust policies will recognise their responsibilities in relation to public policy and legislation. They will detail the procedure for raising a concern and explain the process of investigation. The majority of policies will detail the personnel who may be involved in the investigation. Education providers and service providers recognise that raising a concern can be an uncomfortable and sometimes difficult experience, particularly for students, therefore support may be offered to the individual either through a line manager or pastoral tutor.

Further reading

Association of Directors of Social Services (2005) *Safeguarding Adults: A national framework of standards for good practice and outcomes in adult protection work.* Leeds: ADSS.

Basford, L and Slevin, O (2003) *Theory and Practice of Nursing: An integrated approach.* Cheltenham: Nelson Thornes.

This text offers the reader an insight into the professional issues nurses face and the associated complexities.

Mencap (2012) *Death by Indifference: 74 deaths and counting. A progress report 5 years on.* Available at www.mencap.org.uk.

This is a sobering report detailing the failings of agencies in protecting vulnerable adults with learning disabilities.

Northway, R and Jenkins, R (2013) *Safeguarding Adults in Nursing Practice.* London: Sage/Learning Matters.

This is a comprehensive text on safeguarding that explores in more detail the legislation, governance and policies on safeguarding.

Nursing and Midwifery Council (NMC) (2010) *Raising and Escalating Concerns: Guidance for nurses and midwives.* London: NMC.

Read this in conjunction with accessing the NMC's website and resources on raising and escalating concerns at www.nmc-uk.org.The toolkit provides a range of activities based on scenarios in a variety of clinical settings.

Wheeler, H (2012) *Law, Ethics and Professional Issues for Nursing: A reflective and portfolio-building approach.* Abingdon: Routledge.

This text offers an integrated approach to the application of ethical and legal theories of nursing. It contains a variety of case studies.

Chapter 6
The nurse: accountability and professional regulation

John Unsworth

NMC Standards for Pre-registration Nursing Education

This chapter will address the following competencies:

Domain 1: Professional values

1. All nurses must practise with confidence according to *The Code: Standards for conduct, performance and ethics for nurses and midwives* (NMC, 2008), and within other recognised ethical and legal frameworks. They must be able to recognise and address ethical challenges relating to people's choices and decision making about their care and act within the law to help them and their families and carers find acceptable solutions.

Domain 3: Nursing practice and decision making

7. All nurses must be able to recognise and interpret signs of normal and deteriorating mental and physical health and respond promptly to maintain or improve the health and comfort of the service users: acting to keep them and others safe.

NMC Essential Skills Clusters

This chapter will address the following ESCs:

Cluster: Care, compassion and communication

1. As partners in the care process, people can trust a newly registered graduate nurse to provide collaborative care based on the highest standards, knowledge and competence.

By the first progression point:

1. Articulates the underpinning values of *The Code: Standards for conduct, performance and ethics for nurses and midwives* (NMC, 2008).

Cluster: Organisational aspects of care

9. People can trust the newly registered graduate nurse to treat them as partners and work with them to make a holistic and systematic assessment of their needs; to develop a personalised plan that is based on mutual understanding and respect for their individual situation promoting health and well-being, minimising risk of harm and promoting their safety at all times.

continued . . .

By entry to the register:

20. Acts autonomously and appropriately when faced with sudden deterioration in people's physical or psychological condition or emergency situations, abnormal vital signs, collapse, cardiac arrest, self-harm, extremely challenging behaviour, attempted suicide.

14. People can trust the newly registered graduate nurse to be an autonomous and confident member of the multi-disciplinary or multi-agency team and to inspire confidence in others.

By the first progression point:

1. Works within *The Code* (NMC, 2008) and adheres to *Guidance on Professional Conduct for Nursing and Midwifery Students* (NMC, 2010c).

15. People can trust the newly registered graduate nurse to safely delegate to others and to respond appropriately when a task is delegated to them.

By entry to the register:

2. Works within the requirements of *The Code* (NMC, 2008) in delegating care and when care is delegated to them.

3. Takes responsibility and accountability for delegating care to others.

4. Prepares, supports and supervises those to whom care has been delegated.

17. People can trust the newly registered graduate nurse to work safely under pressure and maintain the safety of service users at all times.

By the first progression point:

1. Recognises when situations are becoming unsafe and reports appropriately.

By entry to the register:

9. Appropriately reports concerns regarding staffing levels and skill-mix and acts to resolve issues that may impact on the safety of service users within local policy frameworks.

Chapter aims

After reading this chapter, you will be able to:

* define the nature and scope of professional accountability;
* demonstrate an understanding of professional self-regulation as it applies to nursing;
* describe how *The Code: Standards of conduct, performance and ethics* (NMC, 2008) can be used to promote safe care, hold practitioners to account and maintain professional standards.

Introduction

This chapter aims to expand on the concept of professional accountability as it applies to patient safety. The nursing profession is under greater public scrutiny than ever before, with major concerns about care provision and the appropriate recruitment and preparation for practice of nursing students (Francis, 2013). Appropriate professional standards already exist and registered nurses are accountable to their patients, their employer, the wider public and the Nursing and Midwifery Council (NMC). This chapter will examine the nature of professional accountability, answering the question 'What is accountability?' It will explore the system of professional self-regulation that exists for nursing and midwifery in the UK, and examine the role and function of the NMC. Throughout the chapter the NMC's *The Code: Standards of conduct, performance and ethics* (2008) will be utilised to illustrate the appropriate standard for practice when making clinical decisions, delegating care to others, raising and escalating concerns and acting without delay when a patient is at risk of harm.

The chapter will explore the nature and scope of professional accountability, accountability to an employer and the role of the professional regulator. Using a series of case studies, based on real-life cases, the issues of accountability for patient safety will be explored and how patient safety issues can be avoided. The first case study will explore early intervention to recognise and respond appropriately to patient deterioration. This case study recognises that failure to rescue is a global problem that accounts for a number of avoidable deaths. The issues related to failure to rescue will be discussed together with an exploration of the various systems that have been put in place to promote more timely recognition and rescue of patients. This section will examine the use of early warning scoring systems and how these can prove useful to practitioners but remain no substitute for sound clinical judgement.

Delegation is a key element of a registered nurse's practice and through a case study and subsequent discussion the chapter seeks to answer the question 'What can be safely delegated to others?' This section will detail the regulator's advice on delegation and the factors that the registered nurse should consider both before delegating care and after the care has been delegated.

Recognising that mistakes do occur, the chapter will examine a medication administration error and the subsequent response to the error. This section will discuss the causes of such errors, how they can be prevented and what action an employer and the NMC may take in such circumstances.

Finally, the chapter examines the issue of raising concerns about standards of care and patient safety and what the registered nurse should and can do if he or she has concerns about care provision. This section illustrates how nurses may be protected by *The Code*, and how and when issues can be escalated if the appropriate response is not forthcoming.

What is accountability?

The NMC's *Code* (NMC, 2008) sets out how nurses and midwives are accountable for acts and omissions in the provision of the care they provide to patients. *The Code* states *as a professional, you are personally accountable for actions and omissions in your practice, and must always be able to justify your decisions* (p2). Professional accountability is an ambiguous term that is open to multiple interpretations (Mander, 1995). The term can mean to be 'counted on' in the sense of being dependable and to be 'counted on' in terms of defending the appropriate standard of care (Bergman, 1981). The NMC describes how accountability is an integral part of practice and that, as a concept, it is fundamentally concerned with professional judgements made in the interests of patients and others in often complex situations (NMC, 2006). Being accountable, registrants (qualified nurses and midwives) must be able to account for the decisions they make. Decision making in professional practice utilises professional knowledge, judgement and skill to decide upon the best course of action for a patient or client.

Accountability takes several forms, with nurses and midwives being professionally accountable to their regulator, the NMC, accountable under contract to their employer and accountable for acts and omissions under the law.

Accountability has four main functions:

- to protect patients;
- to deter practitioners from working outside accepted practice;
- to educate staff;
- to regulate the individuals who make up a professional group.

The exercising of professional accountability by practitioners does provide a degree of protection for patients, in that it promotes practitioners to consider the consequences of their acts or omissions. This process, which involves the use of knowledge, skill and judgement, requires practitioners to weigh up their options and decide upon the best course of action. Considering why the proposed actions are in the best interests of the patient assists in this process and also allows practitioners to learn from clinical reasoning and problem solving.

Most nurses and midwives will have signed a contract of employment in which they will have agreed that they will be accountable to their employer. Under the terms of most contracts the nurse or midwife will be required to work to the employer's policies and procedures. Any deviation from these procedures could be regarded as misconduct by an employer and the employee could be held to account for any such misconduct via the employer's disciplinary procedures. Employers have liability for their employees' acts or omissions and this is called *vicarious liability*. Such liability exists where the employee performs a role or function that the employer requires them to perform, for example a role outlined in the job description. Liability also exists where an employee performs an act that is incidental to employment, such as resuscitating someone who has collapsed and who was a visitor to the hospital. Finally, the employer can also be held liable for acts that the employer is aware the employee performs although such acts may not have been individually sanctioned by the employer (Richardson, 2002).

The final type of accountability is that which relates to the law (Dimond, 2011). Registered nurses are accountable for their actions and omissions under both criminal law (such as prosecutions for assault or under the Misuse of Drugs Act 1974) and under civil law (such as being sued for negligence).

What is professional regulation?

Within the UK most professions are self-regulating. That is, the profession itself sets the standard, monitors compliance and addresses staff who have fallen short of the standard. Self-regulation is seen as the preferred model, as the alternatives such as state regulation are seen as a threat to the status of professions and could lead to state interference in the exercise of professional **autonomy** (Baldwin and Cave, 1999). Self-regulation has been defined as:

> the means by which members of a profession, trade or commercial activity are bound together by a mutually agreed set of rules which govern their relationship with the citizen, client or customer. Such rules may be accepted voluntarily by the profession member or may be compulsory.
> (Better Regulation Task Force, 1999, p3)

Another reason why self-regulation is the preferred model for the professions is that it improves compliance with the rules and standards set by the profession. It is felt that, because the profession itself has set the standard, the members are more likely to work to this standard as it is seen as appropriate to those who are being regulated (Baggot, 2002).

Professional self-regulation is seen as low cost to the state as members of the profession finance the system of regulation through registration fees. While the health professions are regarded as self-regulating, in practice the process is a mixture of self- and state regulation. Most of the professions are directly accountable to Parliament and have to consult with the Privy Council about changes to their roles and functions (Baggot, 2002). This mixture of professional self- and state regulation can lead to tensions from both sides if the Government tries to interfere in professional standards, or when the members of the profession have to pay increasing costs through annual registration fees.

Professional self-regulation has been subject to criticism because of perceptions among the public that the professions act to protect members rather than the public (Baggot, 2002). In addition, the body governing the profession (in the case of the NMC, the Council) may be perceived as lacking legitimacy among the profession itself, with members of the profession resenting having to pay for a body that does not reflect their interests. This resentment has been apparent in nursing at various points since nursing registration was established in 1919 (Davies and Beach, 2000).

Activity 6.1   *Critical thinking*

- Consider what the alternatives are to professional self-regulation, making a list of the pros and cons of each of the alternatives you can think of.

An outline answer is provided at the end of the chapter.

Having explored possible alternatives to professional self-regulation, in the next section we will examine the role and function of the NMC in more detail.

The role and function of the Nursing and Midwifery Council

The NMC is the independent regulator for nurses and midwives in the UK. Established under the 2001 Nursing and Midwifery Order, the organisation is funded predominantly by the fees that nurses and midwives pay to be on the NMC's register. The NMC came into being in 2002 and it is the largest professional healthcare regulator in the world, with responsibility for more than 670,000 nurses and midwives across the UK. The NMC exists to safeguard the health and well-being of the public by ensuring that only those individuals who meet the requirements are allowed to practise as nurses or midwives (NMC, 2012a). The NMC is responsible for:

- maintaining a register of nurses and midwives who are allowed to practise;
- setting the standard for education for entry on to the register of nurses and midwives;
- setting the standards for the conduct and performance of nurses and midwives;
- ensuring that nurses and midwives of the professional register keep their professional knowledge up to date;
- investigating and addressing concerns about nurses and midwives who may be unfit to practise.

The NMC is accountable to Parliament, through the Privy Council, in terms of how the organisation fulfils its responsibilities. In addition, the Professional Standards Authority (formerly the Council for Healthcare Regulatory Excellence – CHRE) is also responsible for reviewing the performance of the NMC and the other UK health and social care regulators (NMC, 2012a).

Protecting the public

The NMC's primary purpose is to protect the public; therefore, as an organisation, the NMC plays a key role in patient safety. While the NMC does not provide care directly to patients, it exerts considerable influence over practitioners and healthcare providers by setting standards for nursing and midwifery practice as well as ensuring that practitioners are, and remain, fit to practise.

The NMC protects the public by setting out various standards, providing guidance, setting out the requirements for entry to the professional register and setting the standards for re-registration. The cornerstone of the professional practice standards produced by the NMC is the NMC's *The Code: Standards of conduct, performance and ethics for nurses and midwives* (NMC, 2008). *The Code*, to give it its shortened title, details the overarching principles that justify the public's trust in the nursing and midwifery professions. It sets out that, to justify such trust, nurses and midwives need to make the care of people their first concern, promote and protect people's dignity, as well as working alongside others (patients and their families) to promote health and well-being. The final overarching principle is that nurses and midwives must be open, honest and act with integrity and that they must uphold the reputation of the profession at all times.

The Code goes on to detail how nurses and midwives must act to ensure that the key principles set out are adhered to. Midwives are required also to adhere to the *Midwives Rules and Standards* (NMC, 2012b), in addition to operating within *The Code*.

In addition to *The Code*, the NMC also issues various standards. You should be familiar with many of these standards as some of them set out the educational course you are following, for example *The Standards for Pre-Registration Nursing Education* (NMC, 2010a). The other main standard relates to *Medicines Management* (NMC, 2007), which sets out in considerable detail all aspects of medicines management from prescribing, supply and storage through to administration and disposal of unwanted medicines.

Finally, the NMC issues guidance on a number of subjects to guide nurses' and midwives' practice. This guidance generally supports elements of *The Code* and illustrates a number of important aspects of practice. Guidance produced by the NMC includes *Record Keeping: Guidance for nurses and midwives* (NMC, 2009) and *Raising and Escalating Concerns: Guidance for nurses and midwives* (NMC, 2010b).

Act without delay

Case study

Victor Hassan is a band 5 registered mental health nurse working on an acute psychiatric ward. Victor has been assigned to care for David Brooks, a 32-year-old man admitted under Section 2 of the Mental Health Act 2007. David is under half-hourly psychiatric observations and Victor is assigned responsibility for these. At 2.00 p.m. David asks Victor if he can visit the next-door ward. Victor assumes this will be all right as David is a frequent visitor to the neighbouring ward where he was an inpatient earlier in the year. Victor asks David to check with Kath Benson, the ward manager, before he leaves the ward.

At 3.30 p.m. David is found in a collapsed state in the day room of the neighbouring ward. He has an empty vodka bottle at his side and, while he is able to open his eyes on command, he appears very drunk and smells strongly of alcohol. Kath instructs staff to take David back to the ward and to call the duty doctor immediately. She asks Victor why David is on another ward and why he has not been undertaking David's half-hourly psychiatric observations.

The doctor attends to assess David and he instructs Kath and Victor to keep an eye on him. Victor continues half-hourly psychiatric observations until the end of his shift and hands over to the next shift, which continues half-hourly psychiatric observations during the night. David is found dead in bed at 7.00 a.m. the following morning.

Activity 6.2   *Reflection*

- Think about the sequence of events that led to David's death. What factors contributed to this tragic outcome?

An outline answer is provided at the end of the chapter.

Having explored the sequence of events in this case study we will now go on to examine in detail how the tragic outcome for David could have been avoided.

The sequence of events in the case study illustrates the 'Swiss cheese' model (Reason, 2000), where all the holes line up to produce the adverse patient safety event. Please refer to Chapter 7, where the 'Swiss cheese' model is explained further. As with many patient safety events, there are numerous opportunities for individuals to intervene to prevent error or to rescue the patient and safeguard his health and well-being. The main issues in the case study are:

- failure to continue psychiatric observations;
- allowing the patient to leave the ward without communicating to colleagues the need for continued observation;
- failure to recognise the risks associated with alcohol intoxication;
- failure to ensure that David's vital signs were monitored;
- inappropriate psychiatric observations during the nightshift, with a corresponding failure to recognise that David had stopped breathing.

The NMC's *Code* (2008) is likely to have been breached by Victor, Kath and other nursing staff in the following ways.

21. *You must keep your colleagues informed when you are sharing the care of others.*

29. *You must establish that anyone you delegate to is able to carry out your instructions.*

32. *You must act without delay if you believe that you, a colleague or anyone else may be putting someone at risk.*

35. *You must deliver care based on the best available evidence or best practice.*

(NMC, 2008, pp4–6)

Failure to rescue

The above case study represents an example of failure to rescue a deteriorating patient. Failure to rescue is an issue of global concern (Clarke and Aiken, 2003; Buykx et al., 2011; Jones et al., 2011), which relates to the failure to prevent patient deterioration arising from a complication of an underlying illness (Silber et al., 1992). Failure to rescue is recognised as a significant issue within acute adult and paediatric nursing. However, as an issue, failure to rescue the deteriorating patient applies across all fields of nursing practice. In 2008 the National Patient Safety Agency (NPSA, 2008a) identified how clients with mental health problems and learning difficulties may also be at risk. The NPSA (2008b) analysed 599 incidents reported through a national reporting and learning system and identified how problems related to rapid tranquillisation, asphyxiation during restraint and choking could lead to medical emergencies. Rapid tranquillisation has been a known risk of death for several years and, despite this, deaths continue to occur (James, 2008).

Nurses are often responsible for continual monitoring and 24-hour care of patients. This places them in a unique position to detect the signs and symptoms of patient deterioration. However, the timely recognition of deterioration and appropriate rescue is a complex process with numerous potential points of failure, including a failure to record observations, a failure to recognise the significance of changes, failures in response and not communicating concerns to other professionals in a timely manner (Haines and Coad, 2001).

In response to the problem of failing to rescue, the National Institute for Health and Clinical (now Care) Excellence (NICE) issued guidance on the recognition of acute illness in hospital patients (NICE, 2007). Alongside this guidance many NHS organisations instituted the use of physiological track and trigger systems (Jansen and Cuthbertson, 2010) and established critical care outreach teams (McArthur-Rouse, 2001).

Early warning score systems

Early warning score (EWS) systems, also known as track and trigger systems, were designed to identify the early signs of patient deterioration (Oakley and Slade, 2006). EWS systems should encourage increased vigilance so that appropriate interventions can be instigated if the patient deteriorates. While the use of EWS systems has become widespread across the NHS, the evaluation of such tools in terms of validity, reliability and utility has not kept pace with their adoption (Cuthbertson, 2003).

EWS systems are not without their critics. One of the major concerns is that there is no standardised system in use across the NHS. Some scores use a combination of single-item and aggregate scores and others use aggregate scores alone (Morgan and Wright, 2007). In addition, there have been concerns that some EWS systems are not sensitive enough, only detecting patient deterioration in some cases as late as 15 minutes before cardiac arrest (Hillman et al., 2005).

In 2012 the Royal College of Physicians developed a new national EWS (NEWS). The NEWS system has been subject to some evaluation but further work is required to test the validity and reliability of the scale. Despite the obvious benefits of a standardised approach, the NEWS system was not immediately adopted across the NHS as uptake has been left to individual NHS organisations.

Within some healthcare settings the availability of equipment to undertake vital observations can be an issue. All healthcare settings, whether mental health, learning disability or nursing homes, should have access to equipment in order to undertake vital observations. Staff should ensure that they are familiar with the equipment available and that they can take and record vital observations and record an EWS. The ability to measure blood pressure using a manual (aneroid) sphygmomanometer is an essential skill for all nurses as overreliance on electronic monitoring equipment can put patients at risk of harm. The NPSA (2007d) identified the need for nurses to be able to record a manual blood pressure because automatic monitors may fail to record or be inaccurate in patients with hypotension.

The above case study represents an example of how *The Code* may be applied retrospectively, after things have gone wrong, to judge the standard of care that should have been provided. In the next section we will look at how *The Code* could assist a registrant to make a decision about whether care can be delegated to others.

Ensuring appropriate delegation of care

Case study

Claire Brown is a band 6 junior ward sister and the link nurse for continence on ward 6, a busy medical ward. She is approached one day by Ben Knight, an experienced healthcare assistant, who has just achieved his NVQ level 4 in healthcare. Ben previously worked on a urology ward in a different NHS Trust, where he was allowed to catheterise men. Ben asks Claire if he might be allowed to undertake male catheterisation on ward 6 in the future. Claire is aware that Ben appears knowledgeable about the procedure and that he is very keen to take every opportunity to expand his role. In the next few months Ben hopes to commence a degree course in nursing if he is able to secure a place at his local university.

Activity 6.3	*Critical thinking*

Think of how Claire might best respond to Ben's request for him to be allowed to undertake male catheterisation.

- Do you think this is a procedure that could be delegated to a healthcare assistant?
- What factors might you need to take into consideration before it was delegated?
- Whom do you think Claire would need to discuss this with before allowing Ben to possibly perform such a procedure?

Outline answers are provided at the end of the chapter.

We will now examine how care can be appropriately delegated to others and what actions a registered nurse must take to ensure that patient safety is maintained.

The NMC's *Code* provides some guidance about the delegation of care to other staff. Specifically, *The Code* outlines how:

29. you must establish that anyone you delegate to is able to carry out your instructions;

30. you must confirm that the outcome of any delegated task meets required standards;

31. you must make sure that everyone you are responsible for is supervised and supported.

(p5)

So the NMC provides some useful generic guidance in terms of identifying whether the delegate (the person to whom the work is being delegated) has the required knowledge and skill to perform the delegated task. It also details how delegates must be supervised by a registered nurse and how the registered nurse should specifically confirm that the delegated care was delivered and whether the desired outcome was achieved. What *The Code* does not provide is specific guidance about the types of care task that can be delegated.

All too often care tasks are delegated on the basis that they are classified as routine by registered nurses. Delegation of tasks such as patient observations, whether vital observations or psychiatric observations, is commonplace, with these tasks often been delegated to the most junior and inexperienced of staff. As outlined earlier in the chapter, these types of observation are not routine and they require a considerable degree of skill, knowledge and judgement in order that they are undertaken safely. Clearly, it would be impossible for every aspect of care to be provided by qualified nursing staff. Indeed, Carr and Pearson (2006) identify how delegation is often driven by one of two imperatives – either pragmatic to ensure that the service can be delivered, or because the delegation promotes more timely care for patients. So this leads to the question 'What can be delegated safely?'

What can be delegated safely?

Outside a hospital setting, it is common to see some relatively complex procedures and care delegated to family members and, in some cases, to patients themselves. This can include mechanical ventilation, care of central venous access devices and intravenous antibiotics. This suggests that even complex care could be delegated to non-registered staff. To some extent, decisions about what aspects of care should be delegated to healthcare assistants rests with the employer, for example the NHS Trust. The employer would, by agreeing to the delegation of the care, be vicariously liable for any act or omission that resulted in harm to the patient.

Delegation involves the allocation of work to another (the delegate) who accepts responsibility for completing the work. Within a professional nursing context the delegator remains accountable for the performance and outcome of the work that has been delegated (Gilien and Graffin, 2010).

Organisational approval aside, the NMC (2012c) states that the decision about whether care should be delegated relates to:

- whether delegation of the care would allow for more timely and continuous care provision;
- whether the performance of the care task can be separated from aspects of clinical reasoning and decision making;
- the stability of the patient;
- whether the outcome, to some extent, is predictable.

So considering Ben's request to undertake male catheterisation, it may be possible to provide him with the skills to undertake the procedure. In certain circumstances male catheterisation, for example 12-weekly routine catheter changes in patients without obstruction, could be delegated to Ben (with organisational approval). However, it would be inappropriate to delegate new catheterisations or urgent catheter replacements because of catheter blockage, as these are not stable patients and the outcome of the procedure is not predictable. In addition, an element of clinical decision making is required in both cases. It would not promote continuous care if the registered nurse is involved in the decision making and the procedure is then performed by another non-registered worker.

Another important aspect of delegation is ongoing supervision and training for the delegate. The Royal College of Nursing (RCN, 2006) emphasises the need for ongoing supervision and clinical advice for support workers taking on delegated roles and how systems must be in place to ensure continued competence and to promote lifelong learning.

In the next case study we will look at a medicines administration error. Earlier in Chapter 4 we examined medicines administration and patient safety in considerable detail. Given that medicines administration errors are one of the most common reasons why registrants are referred to the NMC for impaired fitness to practise, it would be remiss of us to ignore this issue in this chapter. However, the focus in the next case study is on what action the registrant took to safeguard the patient's health and well-being.

Responding to medicines administration mistakes

Case study

Guy Cross is a newly qualified band 5 staff nurse working on a care of the elderly ward. He is busy administering the 10.00 a.m. medicines to patients in one of the bays of the ward. He has just given Mr King his 10.00 a.m. Enalapril 10mg tablet and he has kept Mr King's prescription sheet to one side as he will need to get a second nurse to check out his morphine sulphate tablets (MSTs) 10mg shortly. He tells Mr King that he will bring his MSTs shortly and moves to the next patient. Mr Swinton is the next patient and Guy starts preparing his 10.00 a.m. medicines. The first drug on the prescription sheet is an Enalapril 10mg tablet, which is a common medicine used on the ward. Guy pops the tablet out of the blister pack into a medicines pot. At this point the emergency alarm sounds from a different bay. Guy immediately places the medicines and the prescription sheets into the trolley and locks the trolley, moving it into the corridor as he rushes to assist colleagues with an emergency.

Around 15 minutes later Guy returns to the bay with the medicines trolley. He takes out Mr King's prescription sheet and notices that there is a medicines pot containing Enalapril 10mg. He administers this to Mr King mistakenly thinking that this is the point he was up to with the medicines round when the emergency alarm had sounded. After administration he goes to sign the prescription/medicine record and notices his initials in the box for 10.00 a.m. Guy immediately realises his mistake, but Mr King has already swallowed the second tablet. Guy informs Janet Thompson, the ward sister, and rings the duty doctor for advice. The doctor advises Guy to monitor Mr King's blood pressure and pulse half hourly.

Guy informs Mr King of the error and that he will be monitored closely for the rest of the day and that the doctor will come to review him shortly. Guy completes an incident form about the error.

Activity 6.4 *Critical thinking and reflection*

- What factors led directly and indirectly to the medicines administration error?
- Reflect on how Guy could have prevented this error and what action he might take to ensure no repetition.
- How do you think the Trust and/or the NMC would deal with this error?

Outline answers are provided at the end of the chapter.

In the next section we will examine the causes of error outlined in the last case study and examine what action, if any, Guy's employer and the NMC might take.

The case study highlights a common error in medicines administration in that the wrong drug was given to the wrong patient. What is uncommon in this incident is the fact that the drug is identical for both patients but, by administering it to the wrong patient, Guy has unwittingly overdosed Mr King. There are a number of mitigating factors in this case study, not least the unexpected emergency situation, and this will be discussed in more detail shortly. Guy is professionally accountable for the error in drugs administration and, in this case, his conduct would be judged against the NMC's *Standards for Medicines Management* (NMC, 2007). In this case, Guy would have breached Standard 8, which states:

> *As a registrant, in exercising your professional accountability in the best interests of your patients:*
>
> *– you must be certain of the identity of the patient to whom the medicine is to be administered.*
> (p6)

Despite the error, Guy acted in the best interests of Mr King by immediately disclosing the error and seeking medical review. This action accords with Standard 24 of the NMC's *Standards*, which relates to the management of adverse events:

> *As a registrant, if you make an error you must take any action to prevent any potential harm to the patient and report as soon as possible to the prescriber, your line manager or employer (according to local policy) and document your actions.*
> (p9)

In addition, Guy disclosed to Mr King that the error had occurred, apologised for the error and put in place procedures to prevent or detect harm. This is in keeping with *Being Open when Patients are Harmed* (NPSA, 2005), which requires NHS organisations to disclose when errors that may affect patients' safety have occurred.

One of the key elements of the above case study is that Guy took immediate action to safeguard Mr King's health once he discovered the error. This is an essential part of providing safe care. While we all strive to avoid errors and systems exist to either minimise or design out errors, it is generally accepted that errors will occur (Hughes, 2008). For this reason most organisations adopt a 'no blame' or 'fair blame' approach to medicine errors. No blame policies seek to identify learning from patient safety incidents and then implement safer systems while not blaming individual errors (Wachter, 2012). However, continued errors on the part of a practitioner that are of a similar nature may suggest a lack of competence or a blatant disregard for reasonable standards of patient safety. Such failures may lead to action by the employer or by the professional regulator. It is for this reason that some organisations adopt a fair blame policy. Fair blame encourages openness and learning from errors without the automatic risk of disciplinary action. However, such action can be instigated if repeated errors of a similar nature are reported. Copping (2005) details how open and blame-free approaches to reporting drug-related errors are a prerequisite to safe and effective medicines management.

In light of the fact that the drug administration error from Guy was a single isolated incident with mitigating features and that he took appropriate action to safeguard the patient's well-being, it would be unlikely and inappropriate for him to be disciplined by his employer or for him to be reported to the NMC. Instead, it is likely that the employer would work with Guy to examine the cause of the error and to provide education and advice to him to prevent any recurrence. The NMC, in its *Advice and Information for Employers of Nurses and Midwives* (2011), sets out that misconduct could involve any significant failure to deliver adequate care. When nurses are referred to the NMC, a finding of impaired fitness to practise involves making a judgement about the nurse's previous career, whether the alleged misconduct represents a pattern of behaviour and whether the allegations are easily remedied or have been remedied through training etc. In Guy's case this is a single isolated incident that can be easily remedied through retraining or instruction and reflection on the events that led to the error. Therefore, the medicines administration error that Guy made should not be referred to the NMC.

Using *The Code* to raise concerns

Case study

Julie Carr has been a registered nurse (band 5) for three months. She is one of several band 5 nurses who are on the medical directorate rotation. Julie applied for the rotational post as she felt it was an excellent way to consolidate her experience while she worked in a range of specialties. Julie and three of her colleagues from the rotation have been asked to work on ward 2, a ward that has been specially reopened because of winter pressures. Julie has been on duty for the past three days and the ward is gradually filling up with medical admissions. Julie and her colleagues are concerned that there is no identified ward sister and that all of the six permanent staff on the ward are relatively inexperienced. Yvonne Frame, the Matron, is looking on for the ward and, while Yvonne is very supportive, her other duties mean that she is not readily available to assist staff.

Ward 2 is heavily reliant on bank and agency staff and the rapid increase in the number of patients has resulted in some complaints about patient care and, in particular, about the quality of the record keeping when patients have been transferred or discharged from the ward.

Julie is concerned that something very serious is going to happen and that it is unfair to leave so many inexperienced staff to effectively manage a busy ward.

Activity 6.5   *Critical thinking*

- What do you think Julie should do given the situation she and her colleagues are facing?
- Make short notes about Julie's options and the possible consequences of each course of action.

An outline answer is provided at the end of the chapter.

Raising and escalating concerns is a complex but vitally important area of clinical practice. Without appropriate action by registered nurses and others to address concerns about the environment or care provision, patients will remain unprotected and their safety will be compromised. In the next section we will review the action Julie and her colleagues should have taken to safeguard patient care. We will also explore the use of *The Code* as 'the defender' of care standards.

The last case study illustrates how *The Code* may serve a dual purpose. While *The Code* sets the standards by which practitioners operate, it can also serve as a useful backup when raising concerns about standards of care. Under *The Code* Julie is duty bound to raise concerns about the standard of care on the ward. *The Code* states:

32. *You must act without delay if you believe that you, a colleague or anyone else may be putting someone at risk.*
33. *You must inform someone in authority if you experience problems that prevent you working within this code or other nationally agreed standards.*
34. *You must report your concerns in writing if problems in the environment of care are putting people at risk.*

(NMC, 2008, p5)

In light of the requirements of *The Code* Julie, either alone or preferably collectively with her colleagues, must raise concerns about the lack of leadership and the staffing levels on the ward. These concerns can be raised verbally with the Matron. If they are raised verbally, Julie should maintain a record of the discussions she has had. The concern can also be raised in writing to the Matron and, again, a copy of any correspondence should be retained by Julie. When raising concerns Julie should indicate that she is doing so as required under the NMC's *Code*, citing where possible the sections of *The Code* that she believes are being compromised by the staffing problems.

If Julie fails to raise her concerns she, alongside her nursing colleagues, will be held to account for any failings in the care provided. By raising concerns about staffing and the impact this is having on adherence to *The Code*, Julie is also engaging the accountability of more senior staff within the nursing structure. Maintaining records of any discussions or copies of any letters sent is an important part of raising and escalating concerns. If Julie is subsequently reported by a patient, relative or the Trust to the NMC, she will need evidence that she raised concerns about standards and staffing levels.

If the situation did not improve after initially raising concerns, Julie and her colleagues could seek advice from their professional association, for example the Royal College of Nursing, or trade union, for example Unison. In addition, the NMC's guidance on *Raising and Escalating Concerns* (NMC, 2012d) details how further correspondence should be sent to more senior managers in the Trust if the problem is not resolved. In addition, most Trusts would have a whistleblowing policy that should be followed. If all of this fails to resolve the situation and Julie remains concerned about patient safety, she could report the issues and her attempts to blow the whistle to the Care Quality Commission (CQC).

In most cases the simple act of raising concerns and citing *The Code* will have the desired effect and managers would take action to correct any concerns identified. However, in some situations staff have either failed to take action and/or managers have failed to act on such information, with disastrous consequences for patient safety and for the professional involved. There is no clearer illustration of this than what happened at the Mid Staffordshire NHS Trust (Francis, 2010).

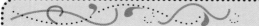

Chapter summary

This chapter has explored the concept of professional self-regulation and accountability. It has sought to illustrate, through a series of case studies, how the NMC's *Code* can be considered as a double-edged sword. On one hand, *The Code* can be used to judge the performance and conduct of a registrant and, on the other, it can prove a useful tool to safeguard both the registrant and patient safety. While the NMC's *Code*, standards and guidance can provide some useful pointers for practice, they tend to be generic and many areas of practice are complex. Therefore, registrants are required to utilise other sources of knowledge and their experience in order to make reasoned decisions about the best courses of action. The important thing when making such decisions is that registrants must be able to offer rationales for their chosen courses of action and, in all cases, the overriding principle of making the care and safety of people their first concern must be evident.

Activities: brief outline answers

Activity 6.1: Critical thinking (page 100)

You may have identified one or more of the following alternatives to professional self-regulation.

*   **State regulation**: This would involve the Government setting standards and deciding who should be allowed entry to the register. Registrants would not pay a fee. Sanctions may be made against registrants who do not meet Government standards or targets.
*   **No regulation**: In theory this could result in anyone calling themselves a nurse or midwife. Local variations in standards of education may make moving between areas in the UK difficult. Not addressing registrants who were unfit or unsafe to practise would place the public at considerable risk of harm.
*   **Local regulation**: Local managers would set standards. Again, considerable variation would exist across the UK and between regions. Scandals such as those at Mid Staffordshire Hospital (Francis, 2010) and Maidstone and Tunbridge Wells NHS Foundation Trust (Healthcare Commission, 2007) have highlighted what can happen when local managers set standards to try to achieve financial balance and targets.

Activity 6.2: Reflection (page 102)

You are likely to have identified some of the following from the sequence of events:

*   failure to ensure that psychiatric observations were conducted;
*   failure to ensure that permission was obtained to visit another ward;
*   not handing over the need for psychiatric observations to the other ward;
*   failure to identify the risks associated with a high alcohol intake;
*   failure on the part of the doctor and the nursing staff to ensure that regular vital observations were taken and recorded;

- psychiatric observations during the night being inadequate as they did not identify that David had in fact died some hours earlier.

Activity 6.3: Critical thinking (page 105)

You are likely to have considered some of the following.

- Ideally, Claire should respond positively to Ben's enthusiasm to develop his skills and knowledge. However, it would be premature to make a full response and Claire should be honest and say that the issue would require some careful thought before it might be agreed.
- The decision about whether the procedure should be delegated would lie with the individual registrant – so, irrespective of whether you agree with others, your decision could be the correct one for you as a future registrant. However, remember that you should have a clear rationale for your decision.
- Ben would need some training and an assessment of his competence to perform the procedure before it could be delegated. In addition, it would be necessary to consider which patients might be suitable before he could undertake the procedure.
- Claire probably needs to discuss the notion of Ben doing the procedure with other nursing colleagues and with her line manager before even contemplating making a proposal to the senior management in the Trust.

Activity 6.4: Critical thinking and reflection (page 107)

- **Source of the error**: While the interruption because of the emergency contributed to the mistake, the medicines administration error is simply that the wrong drug was given to the wrong patient because of a failure to check that the drug had not previously been administered.
- **Prevention**: The error could have been prevented by simply starting again following the interruption and disposing of the medicine already in the medicine pot. To prevent future errors Guy should ensure that he adheres to the five rights of medicines administration (Tyreman, 2010):
  - RIGHT patient;
  - RIGHT drug;
  - RIGHT dose;
  - RIGHT time;
  - RIGHT route.
- **Action by the Trust/NMC**: In order to promote patient safety and timely action following medicine errors the Trust should operate a fair blame or no blame medicines administration policy. As this is a single isolated incident and Guy took immediate action to safeguard the patient, no disciplinary action should take place and referral to the NMC would not be warranted.

Activity 6.5: Critical thinking (page 109)

- **Actions**: Julie and her colleagues should put in writing to their line manager their concerns about patient safety and staffing levels. They should indicate that they are required to do this under the NMC's *Code* and they should request a response to their letter.
- **Possible options**: If the first option is not successful, Julie and her colleagues could consider writing or contacting their trade union or professional organisation. A further letter could be sent to the Director of Nursing or equivalent individual on the Trust Board. Raising or escalating concerns takes a great deal of courage and staff often worry about this having a negative impact on their future careers. However, not raising concerns can also result in damage to an individual's future career as the registrants themselves may end up being referred to the NMC by patients or their relatives. It is possible to raise concerns and remain professional. Using the NMC's *Code* demonstrates that you are genuinely concerned for patients rather than simply intent on making trouble. In addition, presenting possible solutions in any correspondence would go a long way to helping people understand that your intent is to resolve the problem.

Further reading

Caulfield, H (2005) *Vital Notes for Nurses: Accountability.* Wiley-Blackwell: London.

Chapter 11 of this book (page 157 onwards) explores some of the other aspects of professional and ethical accountability particularly around issues related to abortion and palliative care. Reading this chapter will enable you to examine accountability outside the patient safety arena and expand your understanding of *The Code* and professional conduct.

Tingle, J (2004) The legal accountability of the nurse, in Stephen Tilley and Roger Watson (eds) *Accountability in Nursing and Midwifery*, 2nd edition. London: Wiley-Blackwell.

Chapter 5 of this book (page 47 onwards) specifically examines the legal accountability of the nurse and discusses issues such as negligence, dispute resolution, redress and examining some of the scandals that have influenced the development of clinical governance in the NHS. Reading this chapter will enable you to learn more about the legal issues that can affect nursing and to gain a greater understanding of the background to clinical governance.

Useful websites

www.advancedpractice.scot.nhs.uk/legal-and-ethics-guidance/accountability/accountability-to-the-profession.aspx

This is NHS Scotland's Advanced Nursing Practice Toolkit information on accountability.

www.nmc-uk.org/Nurses-and-midwives/Regulation-in-practice

This is the Nursing and Midwifery Council's advice on regulation in practice.

www.rcn.org.uk/development/health_care_support_workers/professional_issues/accountability_and_delegation_film

This will take you to the Royal College of Nursing's guidance on accountability and delegation.

Chapter 7
Human error: systems and human factors in patient safety

continued . . .

By the first progression point:

1. Responds appropriately when faced with an emergency or a sudden deterioration in a person's physical or psychological condition (for example, abnormal vital signs, collapse, cardiac arrest, self-harm, extremely challenging behaviour, attempted suicide) including seeking help from an appropriate person.

By the second progression point:

6. Measures and documents vital signs under supervision and responds appropriately to findings outside the normal range.

9. Undertakes the assessment of physical, emotional, psychological, social, cultural and spiritual needs, including risk factors by working with the person and records, shares and responds to clear indicators and signs.

10. With the person and under supervision, plans safe and effective care by recording and sharing information based on the assessment.

By entry to the register:

19. Refers to specialists when required.

20. Acts autonomously and appropriately when faced with sudden deterioration in people's physical or psychological condition or emergency situations, abnormal signs, collapse, cardiac arrest, self-harm, extremely challenging behaviour, attempted suicide.

21. Measures, documents and interprets vital signs and acts autonomously and appropriately to findings.

Chapter aims

After reading this chapter, you will be able to:

- begin to understand the relationship between technical and human error;
- identify the role that human factors play in error;
- glean an appreciation of the skills you will require to raise concerns if required.

Introduction

Air crash blamed on pilot error . . .
Patient death: human error to blame . . .

This chapter will explore the concept of human error. Most of us will have read newspaper headlines similar to the examples above, but what does this mean? Are they referring to errors caused by one individual or a group of individuals and is the 'blame' justified? We will discuss the meaning of error in relation to patient safety and we will examine some of the human and system factors that can contribute to error. We will be examining case studies and looking at how healthcare is learning lessons from other industries. We will look at the implications for nurses and examine some of the core non-technical skills required by nurses in order to contribute to the patient safety conundrum.

When is an error an error?

Error is the inevitable downside of having a brain!
(WHO, 2010)

Errors are an inevitable part of life. They can happen as a result of the person approach (human error) or the system approach, which can be multifactorial. Human nature means that we are all predisposed to making errors in life, whether errors of judgement or of action. Some errors are unimportant, for example putting the cutlery in the wrong drawer after drying the dishes or picking up the wrong brand of tea in the supermarket. Others can have much worse consequences, such as buying the wrong house, marrying the wrong person or choosing the wrong career, while some errors can have really dire consequences, such as making the wrong decision to pull out in front of an oncoming car, administering the wrong medicine to a patient or removing the wrong limb. Put simply, Reason (1990) has described human error as a deviation between what was actually done and what should have been done. Errors are made by everyone and are not just the domain of the ignorant and incapable. Regardless of experience, intelligence, vigilance or enthusiasm, humans make mistakes. Sometimes an error may only become a perceived error if something detrimental happens that could not have been predicted. For example, a person may swap his shift with a friend to help him out, only to find that the building in which they work catches fire and he is injured, or a person decides to miss the first train and gets on the second one, which is then involved in a fatal accident. These events are unpredictable but the individual may still feel that he or she had made an error.

Human error is routinely blamed for disasters in aviation, on the roads or railways and in the nuclear industry. It is often all too easy for people to point the finger of blame at the pilot of the plane, the driver of the car, the driver of the train or the person in charge of the nuclear plant. However, humans jump to these conclusions without knowing the full facts or appreciating the complexities of such events. While investigations may well reveal that the burden of blame rests with one individual, close analysis can often uncover a series of events leading up to the incident involving a number of individuals, processes, systems and practices. We will begin to examine some of these factors more closely.

Activity 7.1   *Reflection*

- Think about the last few days. Have you made any errors – not related to work? These errors may have been made at home, at university, while shopping, or with your family or friends.
- What types of errors did you make? Rank them in order of importance according to your personal opinion. You may consider some of them to be 'silly' errors, whereas others might be regarded as more problematic.

As this activity is based on your personal experience, there is no answer at the end of the chapter.

Some of the errors we make can be realised immediately, whereas others only come to light much later on. Put simply, errors may occur because of a number of factors, including clumsy psychomotor activity, for example falling over; stress affecting performance; distractions such as noise, intrusion or interruption; lack of knowledge; communication barriers; poor judgement; and, of course, the wisdom of hindsight. Psychologists have invested much time in analysing errors and we will look at these in a little more detail.

Further analysis of error

There is no one absolute definition of error. However, most people and the literature accept that it involves some kind of deviation from the original intention. Although we have considered errors made by us as individuals, there is also much studied and written about organisations and errors in an effort to understand and learn from them.

Classifying errors has been attempted in the literature, predominantly by the discipline of psychology, and is often approached from several different perspectives. Account is often taken of behaviour, psychological processes and contributory factors.

Professor James Reason (2008) has studied and researched the nature of error extensively and suggests that there are four basic elements to an error.

Intention

- Was there an intention to act or was the action involuntary?
- If intended, did the action achieve the desired outcome?
- Were there any slips or lapses in the planning stage?

The action

- Were there any omissions in the action?
- Were there any intrusions?
- Repetitions – were any of the actions repeated?
- Wrong objects – was something different?
- Were the wrong orders given?
- Was there a problem with timing?

Context

Errors may have been influenced by contextual elements such as:

- stress;
- environment;
- distractions.

Outcomes

Errors are categorised according to the consequential outcome. Some may be disregarded as no harm occurred, for example switching on the toaster instead of the kettle. Switching off the wrong engine in an aircraft is more serious and will have obviously disastrous consequences.

It is clear that some of the factors above could be linked to errors that occur in healthcare settings.

Healthcare errors

Although some of the factors listed above may well be linked to errors in care delivery, it is rather difficult to categorise errors in healthcare and, as Vincent (2010) points out, generic classification systems might be useful to researchers, but in healthcare they may be viewed as being too conceptual and abstract.

You have already been introduced to examples of errors that occur in healthcare in previous chapters and so far we do know that some have been linked to:

- planning;
- checking;
- communicating;
- operating;
- judgement;
- patient misidentification;
- information retrieval;
- gaps in knowledge.

Activity 7.2   *Critical thinking*

In Activity 7.1 we asked you to think about some errors that you may have made.

- What factors do you think might have contributed to some of those errors? You may wish to refer to some of the triggers listed above.

As this activity is based on your own experience, there is no answer at the end of the chapter.

You may have thought that identifying and labelling something as an error was straightforward. In actual fact, particularly in healthcare and patient safety, identifying what is and what is not an error can be complex. We sometimes disregard an error if it is inconsequential. Other undesirable outcomes may suggest an error was made but realised only much later.

Case study

Debra, the ward manager, is documenting the care she has carried out for Harry Robinson, a 5-year-old boy who was admitted earlier in the day with an asthma attack. She is tired after a long shift and she thinks she is developing a cold. She writes instructions for the next shift in relation to carrying out observations, monitoring his peak flow levels and supporting him and his mum in the correct use of his inhalers. After she has written two pages, she realises she has made the entry in the nursing notes of Harry Roberts, another child who is recovering from a tonsillectomy. On realising her mistake, she amends the record by drawing a line through her entry, writing 'written in error'. She then signs and dates the entry. She is complying with hospital policy. She then selects the correct notes and proceeds to document care. She informs the next shift of the error.

Debra made an error. She selected the notes belonging to a patient with a similar name. It was her intention to document care in the notes. She did not check to make sure she had the correct notes and there was no alert sticker on both patients' notes warning that there were patients with similar names on the ward. If we consider the context of the incident, Debra was tired and she felt unwell. On realising her mistake she instigated the correct procedure according to local policy. No harm came to either patient so there was no detrimental outcome. Incidents like this are not uncommon and if detected early can be rectified. The incident was probably disregarded.

However, if Debra had not realised her mistake and staff had carried out her instructions on the wrong patient without realising the confusion, the outcome may have been quite different. You may be thinking that surely the staff on the next shift would realise the documented entries did not necessarily relate to a child recovering from surgery. But what if they did not? Would the fault lie with Debra or the staff on the next shift, or both? What about the administrator who failed to put a sticker on the case notes warning of a similarly named patient on the ward? You can see how this error could have potentially been more serious. It also raises the question of who is at fault. Should anyone be 'blamed' or is it a fault in the system? We have already examined some of the issues arising in previous chapters, but we will explore the concept of **human factors** and system failures in more depth.

Professor James Reason led academic research into how human errors combine with system failures to cause accidents. He studied a number of high-risk industries and high-profile incidents. His work is well known and features in much of the literature on safety and risk. He applied his findings to a number of high-risk areas including healthcare. He recognised that errors often occurred as a result of failings in systems and termed failings in systems as 'latent errors'. He designed a metaphoric model to explain his theory known universally as the *'Swiss cheese' model* (Reason, 1997) (see Figure 7.1).

This hypothetical model illustrates how, in any system, there are many levels of defence. In healthcare this could be checklists, medication checks or patient identification. Each level of

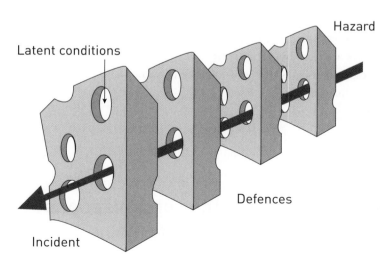

Figure 7.1: The 'Swiss cheese' model (adapted from Reason, 1997)

defence has little holes in it known as **latent conditions**. Examples of these could be lack of training, poor leadership, limited resources or poor communication systems. The presence of latent conditions increases the risk of individuals making active errors, and it is when the latent conditions become aligned over successive levels of defence that they create the potential for a patient safety incident. When an incident does occur it is unlikely that any single action is responsible; it is far more likely that a number of events happened. Some of these may seem minor, but collectively and over a period of time these slips may lead to an incident, even if they have been occurring for some time without any problem.

Activity 7.3   *Reflection*

- In relation to the case study above (Harry Robinson), write down what barriers or latent conditions may have existed that could have led to a potential error.

An outline answer is provided at the end of the chapter.

Each latent condition on its own may seem harmless but it is the cumulative effect that can have potentially serious consequences.

System failures

System failures that have been recognised in healthcare include the following (adapted from Health Foundation, 2011):

- poor communication and unclear lines of authority between nurses, doctors and other professionals;
- reliance on automated systems/technology to prevent errors;
- inadequate methods of sharing information about errors;
- staffing issues;
- cost-cutting measures;
- inconsistent and sometimes fragmented reporting and handover systems;
- presuming others are handling situations;
- medical devices or medicines that look alike/environmental design factors;
- failures in the infrastructure;
- slips and lapses.

You will no doubt recognise that there exists an enormous potential for error considering the stressful and demanding nature of healthcare, but comparison can be drawn with other organisations that have similar factors of stress, pressure and resource issues.

What can we learn from other organisations?

Organisations with a low rate of incidents are termed high-reliability organisations (HROs). HROs are organisations that work in situations that have the potential for large-scale risk and harm, but which manage to balance effectiveness, efficiency and safety. They also minimise errors through teamwork, awareness of potential risk and constant improvement (Health Foundation, 2011). Examples of some of these organisations are the aviation, rail and nuclear power industries. Modern means of transport are increasingly structurally and mechanically reliable; however, significant risks are still abundant, including the threat of terrorism, pilot error, weather and passenger behaviour. When incidents do happen in these organisations, the consequences are usually disastrous and make headline news. Many of you will be aware of disasters such as Chernobyl (1986), where a nuclear reactor exploded, the Piper Alpha oil rig fire (1988), the space shuttle *Challenger* explosion (1986), the *Herald of Free Enterprise* ferry sinking (1987) and the Paddington rail accident (1999). However, incidents like these are rare. The aviation industry, for example, has achieved a very high reliability rate over recent years. There are statistics that indicate we are much more likely to experience an adverse incident if we go into hospital than if we are to fly in an aeroplane. In fact, it is commonly stated that one in ten patients is harmed through healthcare, but this is based on evidence from more than a decade ago and much of it is from outside the UK. Reviewing more recent research suggests that levels of harm range from 3 to 25 per cent in acute care, with a lesser amount of research available in primary care (Health Foundation, 2011). It has been thought for a number of years that many of the techniques and operating systems of HROs could be utilised in healthcare to improve safety and this was at the heart of the report, *An Organisation with a Memory* (OWAM) (DH, 2000a).

Activity 7.4   *Critical thinking*

- What do you think HROs may have in common with healthcare organisations in terms of how they operate and the risks involved?

An outline answer is provided at the end of the chapter.

Key features of high-reliability organisations

Individual authors have different views about the characteristics of HROs but many agree on the following principles.

- Many of these organisations operate in complex physical, social and sometimes political environments.
- The technologies used have the potential for risk and error.
- Consequences of errors could be serious, therefore they cannot use experimentation as a core strategy.
- They use complex processes and systems to manage the way they work.
- There is a good safety culture with leaders and frontline staff taking a shared responsibility.
- There is a focus on checking mechanisms.
- Teamwork is evident.

There are those who dispute that lessons from industry can be translated to healthcare, arguing that healthcare is organic in nature in as much as it deals with humans, most of whom are ill anyway and therefore at increased risk of harm. But if the organisations above carry a high level of risk as to the potential for something to go wrong, it could be argued that healthcare is a high-risk organisation and we should be aiming for a gold standard of 100 per cent in all that we do.

Activity 7.5   *Reflection*

Discuss with a fellow student or mentor: Do you think nurses should always aim to deliver safe care that is of the highest standard, rated at 100 per cent, and settle for nothing less?

- If your answer is yes, is this achievable?
- If your answer is no, discuss why.

As this activity is based on your opinion, there is no answer at the end of the chapter.

If your answer is yes to the above activity, the authors of this book will be pleased to be looked after by you. If your answer is no, we need to consider what is acceptable. But is it that simple?

Maybe you think that achieving 100 per cent safe care is unattainable given the pressures, demands and stressors evident in hospitals and healthcare settings. Maybe you think that 80 per cent safe care is a more realistic goal. If you or a loved one happen to be admitted to the ward that falls into the other 20 per cent quality margin, would you be satisfied?

Imagine if you got on an aircraft to go on holiday and the captain announces 'welcome on board'. During his welcome message he mentions that, due to short staffing and a busy schedule, he will do his best to get you to your destination but he can't guarantee anything! There is every chance you would feel unsafe and probably want to disembark from the aircraft.

The authors of this book suggest that nurses should always strive to achieve 100 per cent safe quality care. The purpose of writing this book is to help equip nurses with some of the skills required to push for quality care and not perpetuate care that is substandard. We will now look at some of these strategies that can be transferred from the above HROs to healthcare.

Strategies to promote safer care

What systems, practices and behaviours can we take from the above HROs to improve safety in our own organisation? Many authors have studied this and the literature reveals that some of the key components in HROs appear to involve discipline, standardisation and teamwork. Organisational learning is also an important feature of HROs. In nursing and medicine some of these components are certainly in existence, but it could be argued that there are inconsistencies and they only come into play at certain times.

Scenario

While the selection and procurement of many healthcare products have been streamlined, it is not uncommon to work with individual doctors who have personal preferences for certain products and devices. Imagine you are working with Doctor Smith, who 'prefers' dressing A to be used on his patient's surgical wound, whereas Dr Evans will not hear of it and insists on using dressing B. Or staff nurse Amy, who always performs an aseptic dressing technique 'this' way, while staff nurse Barbara likes it done 'that' way. This can lead to confusion for nurses, particularly student nurses. All of these professionals may be applying evidence-based practice but tailoring the activity to their own preferences. However, some activities are based on custom and practice. You may need to consider how you would critically analyse this situation. You should now be starting to consider how you would challenge your supervisors in practice to ascertain what is best practice in a non-confrontational way. You may also need to consider how you would approach members of this interdisciplinary team to discuss this. Of course, care should be tailored to the needs of the individual patient and nurses as well as doctors should be exercising their clinical decision-making abilities and professional judgement in each situation. It is perhaps the lack of clear communication that may lead to issues in care.

The NHS is committed to finding new and innovative ways to reduce harm and improve patient safety, much of them learned from HROs. It is in its interests to do so because of the resultant human cost of error. But the NHS also has to consider and manage the resource and financial cost of mistakes. There are a number of programmes, pilots and strategies in place to help staff to achieve this. They are also constantly developing and changing. This book will refer to some of these programmes, some of which you may be familiar with or have heard about. No doubt, by the time of publication, there will be further programmes and strategies implemented. The key message here is to be aware of what current strategies are being rolled out in your placement/ place of employment and to keep abreast of change.

Activity 7.6   *Evidence-based practice and research*

- Find out what patient safety programmes/strategies are being implemented in your own clinical area. You could begin by asking your mentors, searching the Trust intranet for news bulletins or reading policy documents etc.

Use some of the websites at the end of this chapter to assist you in your search.

As this activity is based on your own clinical area, there is no answer at the end of the chapter.

Remember, one of the key features of promoting a safety culture is to ensure that all members of the team are aware of the organisational goals in patient safety. This includes you as a registrant and also as a student.

Human factors

The human factors approach to improving patient safety is gaining great momentum in the UK. 'Human factors' is essentially an umbrella term that encompasses all those factors that can influence people and their behaviour. In a work context, human factors are the environment, organisational and job factors, and individual characteristics that influence behaviour at work (Patient Safety First, 2010a). Focusing on human factors can lead to improvements in day-to-day clinical operations through an appreciation of the effects of teamwork on human behaviour and application in a clinical setting (Clinical Human Factors Group, http://chfg.org/what-is-human-factors). Putting it simply, human factors can be thought of as a concept for designing things in order to make them easy for people to use and help people do the right thing.

The concept of human factors was born out of the twentieth century and is attributed to the military, particularly during the Second World War. The premise is that the design of the workplace, equipment and ways in which we work should be based on human characteristics and abilities – how we process information, communicate, make decisions and remember things – rather than expecting people to adapt to the poorly designed world around them (Norris et al., 2012). However, as well as practical and technical skills such as catheterisation, venepuncture and performing observations, healthcare professionals also need non-technical skills. Non-technical skills are the cognitive and social skills that complement workers' technical skills. Flin et al. (2008) identify these skills and discuss seven: situation awareness, decision making, communication, teamwork, leadership, managing stress and coping with fatigue.

If we consider the people who are represented at the centre of care delivery, these include patients, carers, loved ones, healthcare professionals providing direct care and also those who are indirectly involved in care, such as administration staff, estates, catering, medical device manufacturers, pharmaceutical staff and many others. It is a fact that all of these individuals have the potential to compromise the safety of patients as there is dependence on their competence, abilities, knowledge bases and behaviour. In addition to personnel, healthcare involves the operating and handling of a range of equipment and devices. In order to use equipment correctly we need to understand how things work and how humans make errors.

Designing for simplicity

Standardising design is known to reduce the probability of errors. For example, drugs packaged in similar containers with similar labels have been changed in an effort to avoid mistakes. Standardisation of the single telephone number 2222 for calling resuscitation teams has been implemented in England and Wales. Some syringe drivers have been at the centre of errors as a result of programming variations and steps have been taken by manufacturers to avoid this in the future. Refer to the NPSA website to explore other initiatives that are being implemented constantly. More and more effort is being made to involve users in design. If users are involved in the design process, there is more likelihood that the end product will reflect users' capabilities and understanding and make for a more user-friendly environment that in turn may help to reduce errors. There are those who advocate that manufacturers should always design for the most vulnerable, weakest or least able user, because satisfying their requirements will usually ensure that all others are included (Norris, 2009).

Designing for safety

For systems to work safely, consideration needs to be given to the environment in which patients are cared for. Workplaces should be designed to minimise travel distance and should be designed to meet the needs of all those who use them. There should be space to work that is free from distractions, noise and excessive temperatures. Devices should be user friendly and have alarms that only go off when a response is required; it is all too easy to ignore annoying alarms on machines that appear to be so sensitive that they are almost constantly going off, increasing the temptation to silence them! How many people do you see reading an instruction manual? The layout and storage of equipment should be neat, easy to access and consistent so that staff become familiar with it.

Thinking for safety

All healthcare professionals should be aware of risk and safety issues whatever their role or status. In order to achieve this, individuals must have the cognitive abilities to know how things are expected to work, and to recognise what affects our ability to think and make decisions. We require social and interpersonal skills to help us communicate, challenge, take risks and work collaboratively.

Reliance on memory and the impact of error traps

We know that the human brain is very powerful, flexible and good at finding shortcuts, filtering information and interpreting things. However, it can only have a limited number of things at the forefront at any one time and sometimes it can play tricks on us.

As humans, we need to be aware of some of the error 'traps' that exist. Busy schedules and distractions can interfere with our perception of objects and events. Sometimes we see what we expect to see. This is known as *involuntary automaticity*.

Activity 7.7 **Critical thinking**

Complete the following as quickly as you can:

- What kind of a tree grows from an acorn? (oak)
- What do you call a funny story? (joke)
- What rises from a bonfire? (smoke)
- What is another name for a cape? (cloak)
- What kind of noise does a frog make? (croak)
- What do you call the white of an egg? ( )

How many of you answered the last question as yolk? The correct answer is albumen, but the answer is prompted by the number of oak sound 'primes'. This is one example of our brains being tricked. To illustrate this with more examples, search the internet for optical illusion sites and test yourself!

In the healthcare setting, examples of traps could be setting up an infusion pump that is calibrated in millilitres per day rather than millilitres per hour or vice versa. Other examples are medication packaging that looks the same, resulting in the wrong drug being administered.

When we have a large number of tasks to do, lists can be helpful. We have already discovered this with the WHO Surgical Safety Checklist. Other strategies, such as large whiteboards with tasks or prompts placed in physically accessible places are proven to be useful.

Human factors and teams

There is now greater emphasis on nurses and allied health professionals developing their knowledge through higher education, which has always been present in medicine. The mark of a good nurse has always been to demonstrate care and compassion, empathy and understanding. Nurses have not always been recognised for their academic and intellectual abilities. Arguably, nurse education in the first half of the last century was more focused on doing rather than thinking. In fact, it wasn't a desirable thing to have too many nurses who were highly educated in case they challenged the doctors who predominantly gave them orders. Today, nurses require academic as well as practical skills in order to carry out their work effectively. They also require skills of effective and assertive communication as well as good leadership skills in order to work effectively and safely in multidisciplinary teams.

We know, however, that there exists a reluctance for some to challenge perceived hierarchy. Air crash investigation has revealed that the steepness of professional hierarchy was the cause of some high-profile air accidents. The Tenerife Airport disaster of 1977 is a chilling reminder of this. Two jumbo jets collided on the runway resulting in the horrific deaths of 583 people. The subsequent investigation revealed that the experienced captain had attempted to take off from a foggy runway without permission. The co-pilot and flight engineer were heard on the voice recorder telling the captain that they had not received permission and that there was another aircraft on the runway. The captain did not take any notice of this information from his subordinates.

Activity 7.8   *Reflection*

- Discuss with a registered colleague whether you as a student or your colleague as a registrant believe you are always listened to by other healthcare professionals.

As this activity is based on your own feelings, there is no answer at the end of the chapter.

Some of you may have discussed situations where you felt you were not listened to or were dismissed. Some of you hopefully will have experienced a positive reaction to any concerns raised. Can you begin to make sense of this in terms of behaviours, culture and hierarchy?

Although anecdotal evidence based on our own experience and that of our students and colleagues suggests that **paternalistic** and **hierarchical** attitudes are changing, there is no doubt that they still exist to some degree in some working teams.

Let us now consider the following case study, a very poignant and stark reminder of the role human factors play in healthcare. You can view a video detailing the reconstruction of this case at www.institute.nhs.uk/safer_care/general/human_factors.html. See also Harmer (2005).

Case study

Mrs Elaine Bromiley, a 37-year-old mother of two young children, was admitted for surgery to a clinic in 2005. She required routine surgery to her nasal passages and was considered to be in good health with no significant premorbid history. There were a number of healthcare professionals present in the operating theatre as you would expect: surgeon, anaesthetist, nurses and operating department practitioner, with a further anaesthetist joining the team when it became apparent that there was a problem. All of these people were highly experienced and technically competent professionals. Anaesthesia commenced and the anaesthetist proceeded to insert a laryngeal mask airway into the patient's pharynx. However, it became apparent that this routine procedure was proving difficult and the anaesthetist was unable to insert the device. He also attempted to insert an endotracheal tube, which was unsuccessful and meant it was not possible to ventilate the lungs. This situation is not improbable but it is rare. Consequently, Mrs Bromiley's oxygen saturations fell below normal levels compromising her safety. The medical staff continued to attempt to intubate Mrs Bromiley, recognising the medical emergency. This went on for several minutes. In the meantime one of the nurses made a tracheostomy set available and another booked a bed on the Intensive Care Unit (ICU). However, these actions were overlooked by the medical staff who were still attempting to intubate. Mrs Bromiley's oxygen saturation remained extremely low (less than 40 per cent) for more than 20 minutes. Eventually a decision was made to abandon the procedure and allow the patient to wake up naturally. She was transferred to ICU but by the time her oxygen levels were corrected she had suffered irreparable brain damage and she died two weeks later.

If you have watched the video of this event, you will have observed a number of human factors unfolding. The subsequent detailed investigation highlighted some of these factors, as follows.

- **Teamwork** – there was no clear leader in this situation and no one was taking control. There appeared to be poor coordination with the medical staff all providing help and support, but there was a breakdown in the decision-making process.
- **Communication** – there appeared to be poor communication between the nurses and medical staff. This could have been exacerbated by the perception of authority and hierarchy within the team.
- **Culture** – the nurses knew what to do; they made a tracheostomy set available and booked a bed on the ICU, but they did not speak up when these were not utilised – they didn't know how to broach the subject.
- **Loss of situational awareness** – the medical staff all realised the seriousness of the situation and became focused on repeated attempts to insert the breathing tube, but in doing so lost track of time.
- **Perception and cognition** – actions were not in line with emergency protocol. While many options were being considered under immense pressure, in hindsight they were not the best options.

The aim of the independent enquiry was to establish how and why things went wrong. Ultimately, the staff caring for Elaine Bromiley were competent and not neglectful. They did, however, lose situational awareness and lacked an appreciation of human behaviour under stress. In summary, we can see that some of the human factors that increase risk include stress, distractions, workload, environment, teamwork, leadership, communication and culture.

The above high-profile case has made a huge impact in promoting human factors training and awareness in the healthcare arena. Its importance as a lesson to us all in healthcare is made possible by Mrs Bromiley's husband, an airline pilot and founder and Chair of the Clinical Human Factors Group:

so that others may learn and even more may live.

What can help me as a nurse?

It is important that you raise concerns and 'speak up' if you are worried about something. If it doesn't 'seem' right then chances are it probably isn't. In the case study above, the nurses knew what to do but they were not sure how to speak up and be heard. We acknowledge that, for some, this can be easier said than done and is often dependent on the context of the situation. This is where nurses need to develop professional, effective and assertive communication skills. Raising concerns does not have to be confrontational, challenging or negative. We have already explored the concept of whistleblowing and raising concerns in Chapters 5 and 6. The issue of raising concerns is increasingly being recognised and there are strategies being developed to address the problem.

Communication strategies

We know that inadequate verbal and written communication is recognised as being a common root cause of errors. We know too that there are barriers to communication in teams, including hierarchy, gender, cultural differences and communication styles. In order to address this, some HROs have already adopted alert phrases that appear in their operational procedure manuals and are consistently used and universally understood by staff.

In healthcare, one example of a communication tool that is becoming widely implemented is *SBAR*. This tool originated from the US Navy and was adapted for use in healthcare by Dr M Leonard and colleagues from Kaiser Permanente, Colorado.

SBAR is an abbreviation for:

- **S**ituation
- **B**ackground
- **A**ssessment
- **R**ecommendation.

SBAR is an easy-to-remember mechanism that can be used to frame communications, either verbal or written (Institute for Innovation and Improvement, 2008; see Figure 7.2). The aim of

SBAR is to prevent vagueness, ambiguity and assumption in communication. It is also designed to remove the hierarchy between doctors and others by lifting barriers and providing a common language for communicating critical events. It can be used in a number of situations, handovers, telephone communications and emails.

Situation

- Identify yourself and your location.
- Identify the patient by name and provide a reason for your communication.
- Indicate your reason for calling/concerns.

Background

- Indicate reason for patient's admission.
- Explain significant medical history.
- Provide any relevant information such as diagnosis, medical health, allergies, diagnostic results, medications etc.

Assessment

- Clinical information such as vital signs.
- Other significant observations.
- Your concerns and interpretations.

Recommendation

- Explain what you require from the person you are speaking to and be specific about time-frame.
- Offer suggestions.
- Clarify expectations.

Read back to make sure you have conveyed the message you intended and that it has been understood.

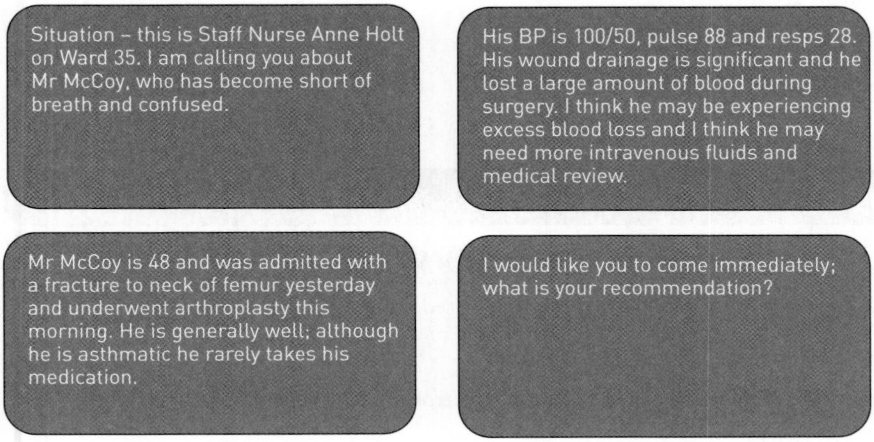

Situation – this is Staff Nurse Anne Holt on Ward 35. I am calling you about Mr McCoy, who has become short of breath and confused.

His BP is 100/50, pulse 88 and resps 28. His wound drainage is significant and he lost a large amount of blood during surgery. I think he may be experiencing excess blood loss and I think he may need more intravenous fluids and medical review.

Mr McCoy is 48 and was admitted with a fracture to neck of femur yesterday and underwent arthroplasty this morning. He is generally well; although he is asthmatic he rarely takes his medication.

I would like you to come immediately; what is your recommendation?

Figure 7.2: SBAR example

Remember, speaking up in the face of a potential breach of patient safety is everyone's business rather than the responsibility of the few (Bromiley and Reid, 2012). It does not matter what field of nursing you are working in and it applies to any situation in which a patient or colleague is vulnerable or at risk.

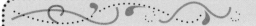

Chapter summary

We have examined the nature of error and the impact that human factors and non-technical skills have on patient safety. We have unravelled some of the differences between individual error and systems error. Ultimately, we have attempted to deliver the hard-hitting message that everyone should have the courage to speak up.

Activities: brief outline answers

Activity 7.3: Reflection (page 120)

You may have identified the following potential latent conditions.

- The individual nurse was tired and unwell and was at the end of a long shift.
- The medical record system failed to identify same name patients.
- The handover/communication system may have been weak.

Activity 7.4: Critical thinking (page 121)

HROs and healthcare organisations may have the following in common:

- high-risk activity;
- complex operating systems;
- systems and processes;
- discipline;
- teamwork;
- financial constraints;
- quality/improvement agenda;
- learning culture;
- serious consequences of error;
- highly trained personnel.

Further reading

Flin, R, O'Connor, P and Crichton, M (2008) *Safety at the Sharp End*. Farnham: Ashgate.

This book focuses on the non-technical skills of personnel based at the sharp end of organisations.

Reason, J (2008) *The Human Contribution*. Farnham: Ashgate.

This is an interesting exploration of human contribution to error in high-risk organisations.

Useful websites

www.chfg.org

Learn more here about human factors at Clinical Human Factors Group.

www.health.org.uk

The Health Foundation is a charity committed to improving healthcare and provides information and research scans on particular topics.

www.institute.nhs.uk

The Institute for Innovation and Improvement provides publications, training resources and toolkits for improving standards and quality in healthcare. It also offers a useful information guide on SBAR.

www.patientsafetyfirst.nhs.uk

This site describes initiatives in patient safety.

Chapter 8
Measuring patient safety and satisfaction

NMC Essential Skills Clusters

This chapter will address the following ESCs:

Cluster: Care, compassion and communication

1. As partners in the care process, people can trust a newly registered graduate nurse to provide collaborative care based on the highest standards, knowledge and competence.

By entry to the register:

8. Demonstrates clinical confidence through sound knowledge, skills and understanding relevant to field.

Cluster: Organisational aspects of care

16. People can trust the newly registered graduate nurse to safely lead, co-ordinate and manage care.

By entry to the register:

3. Bases decisions on evidence and uses experience to guide decision making.

18. People can trust the newly registered graduate nurse to enhance the safety of service users and identify and actively manage risk and uncertainty in relation to people, the environment, self and others.

By entry to the register:

9. Reflects on and learns from safety incidents as an autonomous individual and as a team member and contributes to team learning.
11. Assesses and implements measures to manage, reduce or remove risk that could be detrimental to people, self and others.
14. Works within policies to protect self and others in all care settings including the home care setting.

Chapter aims

After reading this chapter, you will be able to:

- recognise how difficult it is to measure safety;
- identify how safety is currently measured and the importance;
- explore some of the drivers behind measuring safety;
- understand how to apply measurement of safety to practice.

Introduction

NEWS HEADLINE – How safe is our care!

An increase in the expected number of inpatient deaths at a local hospital has raised concerns as to the safety and quality of care delivery. A thorough investigation and inquiry have been requested by the public.

The purpose of this chapter is to raise your awareness and increase your understanding of how difficult it is to measure care that is free from causing harm. Identification and measurement of events that can cause harm to patients in our care are central to patient safety. We will consider some of the different ways in which we measure safety in healthcare, acknowledging that there are strengths and limitations to the range of approaches available. Presently, there is no one single method or approach that can measure the safety of patients in our care. We know that data is rarely cross-referenced across organisations, units or departments, and the assessment of any success in relation to improvement efforts and initiatives becomes almost impossible to measure. We will think about how patient complaints are used to measure satisfaction and how complaints handling is currently under review. We will look at how the NHS Safety Thermometer 'improvement tool' is working towards establishing a baseline to track quality improvement. Measuring is critical to improving quality and ensuring that the patients we care for are safe, but we also know that measuring safety in healthcare is challenging.

Activity 8.1   *Reflection*

- Consider what we measure in our everyday lives and jot down some ideas to think about while you read the following text.

There is no answer at the end of the chapter, but read on for some ideas.

As one possible example, when we cook or bake it is very important that we accurately measure all the ingredients. If we add one more egg to the mixture than is required, we can expect that the end product will be far from satisfactory and the quality will be compromised.

A recipe requires precision and accuracy in order for the end product to be of a satisfactory standard. Measuring safety in healthcare is so much more difficult and we cannot possibly provide the same level of precision. No two situations in healthcare are ever the same; they might be similar but not identical. That is where 'measuring' becomes complex, as it is not clearly defined like the ingredients within a recipe.

If we consider another everyday situation, for example going to the dentist, there are certain 'measures' that we would need to take into account for us to arrive at the dentist on time. Some of these measures we can predict, such as the distance from our house to the dentist. What is a little more difficult to predict is how long it might take to get there. We can plan our route, we can choose a mode of transport, we can estimate the time that it would take to get there, but what we cannot predict is an unexpected situation. You could leave your house only to find that your car has a flat tyre, so you go to the bus stop and have to wait 15 minutes for the next bus. When you eventually get on the bus you are delayed further by roadworks, adding time to your overall journey. All these unexpected events mean that you arrive 30 minutes late for your scheduled appointment.

There are several more 'variables' in the second example than there are in the first. The first example is much more concrete in terms of measurement and precision. The second example is less concrete and more complex in terms of measuring. Although the process of getting to the dentist from your home was similar to your previous visit it was not the same, as you arrived 30 minutes late.

Measuring safety in healthcare is much like the second example – less concrete, more complex, and with numerous variables to consider.

What we do know is that measuring safety is much more complex than measuring out ingredients when cooking or baking, in terms of quality. Wherever we provide care we are constantly being told to count and report, but little is known about how organisations actually go about it. Different organisations, units and departments collect information in very different ways, which means that comparisons across these areas can become meaningless. Measuring healthcare outcomes is complex and difficult.

Why measuring matters

Safety measurement in healthcare has mostly been based on the number of past events that have caused some sort of harm to the patients we care for. Over the past ten years we have seen healthcare flooded with data and statistics on medical error and harm caused to the patients that we care for. Some of the harm that has been caused has been catastrophic, demonstrating healthcare failure and a decline in public confidence and trust in healthcare delivery. We know that we need to make healthcare safer. Among a growing number of major Government reports, professional reports and reviews it becomes increasingly difficult to identify the concepts and technical features of safety that we actually need to measure.

The publication of the report *An Organisation with a Memory* (OWAM; DH, 2000a) focused attention on measuring harm caused to patients and learning from mistakes and errors. Several initiatives have followed, for example *Saving Lives* in 2005 (replaced by DH, 2007). Despite this, more than 13 years after OWAM, it is difficult to know whether patients are any safer in the NHS than they were, particularly in light of the Mid Staffordshire public inquiry and other tragic cases of healthcare failure. We have already recognised that measuring the harm that we can cause to patients in our care is not straightforward and that it is in fact multidimensional. Our inability to determine whether healthcare systems are safer is partly due to a lack of universal clarity over what we actually need to measure. What we currently measure is not how safe healthcare systems are now, but how harmful they have been in the past. Safety is dynamic, fluid and ever changing in healthcare delivery and that is what makes it so difficult to measure.

Mortality rates as a measurement and indicator of quality and safety

Some claim that measuring the number of deaths in a particular Trust or organisation is an indicator as to how safe care is. Mortality rates are risk-adjusted, which means that they take into consideration factors that could increase the likelihood of death. There are over 300 different variables that hospitals need to provide, covering issues such as age, time of diagnosis, lifestyle and existing illnesses. The problem in relation to how accurate this information is relies very heavily on compiling and interpreting those 300 different variables. What we need to recognise is that this cannot be an exact science with so many variables; accuracy becomes very dependent on the information being submitted properly. It is not unheard of for data to be submitted incorrectly or not at all.

Activity 8.2   *Reflection and critical thinking*

Consider the previous paragraph in relation to the following.

In the 1860s Florence Nightingale noted that 'average mortalities' tell us about the percentage of people that will die in any one year:

> *We know, say, that from 22 to 24 (people) per 1,000 will die in London next year.*
> (Nightingale, 1860/1969, p124)

She then goes on to mention that we should question why we are actually recording such information if we are not prepared to act upon or change our practice to promote better health and safer care:

> *It is not for the sake of piling up miscellaneous information or curious facts, but for the sake of saving life and increasing health and comfort.*
> (p125)

- In healthcare today, do you think that we still measure and collect information purely for the 'sake' of it, or do you think that it is used to save lives and influence the safety agenda?
- Have we really moved forward?

It might be useful to share your thoughts with your practice mentor.

As this activity is for your own reflection, there is no answer at the end of the chapter.

If we look at mortality rates linked to children's heart surgery in Leeds at the beginning of 2013, all surgery was stopped because concerns were raised over a high number of deaths. A week later this suspension was lifted as a detailed investigation revealed that crucial information was missing, which skewed the overall picture. One simple piece of information that was needed was the weight of the baby that was having the operation, but the weight was missing in 35 per cent of the cases. This meant that the data was very poor quality and gave the impression that the death rate for children having heart surgery was high. Once again, we find ourselves in a position where measuring safety and quality is difficult, but also public confidence is lost as people struggle to come to terms with the fact that healthcare can be a 'risky business'.

Some believe that mortality rates are a good indicator as to how well a Trust or organisation is performing, while others remain sceptical, suggesting that it is very much dependent on good-quality measuring and data collection. One message that is clear is that, even though mortality rates are not perfect, they are a sign that something might be wrong and should definitely not be ignored.

Activity 8.3   *Reflection and critical thinking*

It might be useful to try to find information about mortality rates within your own Trust or organisation. Discuss where you would find this information with your practice mentor.

You might want to look at:

www.drfosterhealth.co.uk/
http://myhospitalguide.drfosterhealth.co.uk/

The information provided by Dr Foster is available to the public.

*   How might this information and data inform the public?
*   Could the public make decisions on where they want to receive treatment and care, based on this information and data?
*   Do you think that the public should expect the same standard of treatment and care in every Trust and organisation?

As this activity is for your own reflection and critical thinking, there is no answer at the end of the chapter.

We have considered mortality rates as a measure in terms of overall performance within a Trust or organisation; however, there are other ways to measure safety and quality.

Measuring to improve safety and quality

In 2010 the NHS Outcomes Framework was published (DH, 2010b), and afterwards two further frameworks, the most recent being for 2013/14. These frameworks contain key factors to help the healthcare system to focus on measuring health outcomes, moving away from process targets. Some process targets have been blamed for distorting clinical priorities, for example the four-hour target for waiting times in A&E has led to holding patients requiring immediate attention and care in trolley waiting areas. This could be considered as manipulating the situation so that process targets are met.

Activity 8.4 *Reflection*

Below is an example of a process target taken from the news in June 2013:

NHS 'misses' A&E waiting time target. A total of 313,000 patients waited more than four hours, up 39% on the similar period in 2012. That represented 5.9% of patients when the NHS is only allowed leeway of 5% – the worst performance in nine years.

- Consider this information in light of your own experiences.
- Consider what might be measured in order to produce these numbers and statistics.

As this activity is for your own reflection, there is no answer at the end of the chapter.

Process targets can put enormous strain on the people who provide healthcare services. Staff work very hard to meet the process targets, but sometimes the targets that have been set become more and more difficult to achieve as demands on the service become greater and resources dwindle. This can be very demoralising for staff, but patients have also come to expect that their needs will be met within a certain timeframe. On the occasions when process targets are 'breached' or not met, patients more often than not will raise their concerns or complain.

Patient complaints as a measure

Another indicator that is used to measure safety and the care experience is patient complaints. Patient complaints are well recognised as a measure of dissatisfaction that can arise from elements of the care experience that did not meet patients' expectations, preferences or goals.

Patient complaint data can contribute to clinical care improvement strategies. A link between measuring patient complaints or dissatisfaction and patient safety can be made, but once again difficulty arises from what it is that we actually need to measure. Individual patient satisfaction might be influenced by many variables. We have already noted that, in relation to mortality rates, 300 variables need to be considered. The more variables we consider the less accurate the data collection process becomes.

Activity 8.5 *Critical thinking*

- How can we capture and measure patient satisfaction?
- Think about some of the many variables you would need to consider if you were trying to measure patient satisfaction/dissatisfaction? It might be useful to write your thoughts down.
- Consider how difficult it would be to measure satisfaction if the patient was very ill, elderly or confused. Would patients falling into these categories be classed as 'unable to participate'?

Outline answers are provided at the end of the chapter.

What we must also consider when trying to measure patient satisfaction is whether the data that is collected reflect the care journey as a whole, or just a fraction or part of the care experience that did not meet the patients' preferences, expectations or goals. Patient satisfaction would again appear to be one of those difficult concepts to measure effectively, but there is evidence to suggest that problem areas in healthcare delivery can be identified, service improvements made and policies influenced.

It is also worth noting that the work of the NHS complaints system in England is currently under review. Patient experience has a much greater influence and impact than ever before, on how healthcare providers and commissioners work and on how money is distributed and moved around the healthcare system. It is evident that we must involve patients and listen to their concerns so that we can act accordingly to improve the care that we deliver. It is well documented in the Francis Report (2013) that there was a lack of responsiveness to complaints made by patients and relatives. As a result of the inquiry, 13 recommendations have been made that directly relate to complaints and their handling. Eight areas for consideration, specifically relating to the handling of complaints and concerns, have been identified within the terms of reference of the review. The Royal College of Nursing (RCN) is also actively involved in this review and will be offering a formal response.

Case study

47 Entwhistle Street
Somewhere Nearby
SN01 1DR
16.09.13

Dear Chief Executive,

I am writing to you because I feel that I have nowhere left to go with my complaint. Nobody seems to want to take any responsibility for what happened to me when I was admitted to hospital. Although I don't want to cause any trouble, I do feel that someone needs to take the matter seriously so that it doesn't happen to someone else, perhaps more vulnerable than I was at the time. My recovery and subsequent return to work have been delayed by a number of months due to the impact of what I believe to be a lack of competence.

To date, I feel that there has been no acknowledgement of the mistakes that were made. There would appear to be failure at all different levels within the Trust to actually understand what it is that I am complaining about. I have yet to receive a response in writing to my complaint and the verbal responses that I have received are not proportionate to the seriousness of my complaint. I feel like I am 'banging my head against a brick wall' and that I am being treated as just a joke.

I am not looking for a financial remedy; all I really want is an apology and reassurance that the mistakes made will not happen again. I am writing to you out of desperation and to request that my complaint is fully explored and investigated. If I do not receive any response, or receive an inappropriate one, I will be left with no choice but to take this matter further.

continued . . .

> The reference number for my complaint is REF: 12453. I do not have the inclination or the time to explain the nature and specifics of my complaint again. I'm worn out by the whole process now and I'm beginning to think that people are hoping that I will just drop it, or forget about it. I'm not prepared to do that and that is why I am writing to you.
>
> I look forward to hearing from you.
>
> Yours faithfully,
>
> Peter Piper

If we look at Peter Piper's complaint it is obvious that there has been a lack of response. He clearly feels that his complaint has not been taken seriously and the only option that he felt he had was to write to the Chief Executive of the Trust before taking his complaint further. It is important that we acknowledge complaints and handle them appropriately. If we handle complaints promptly we can work towards a resolution, improve services and prevent the same mistake happening again. When we are unable to achieve this, the complainant, whether that is a patient or a relative, looks for an alternate remedy.

The role of the Parliamentary and Health Service Ombudsman

We know that the NHS and other organisations provide excellent care on a daily basis to thousands of people. We also know that at times mistakes are made and things do go wrong. When this happens, how organisations and people deal with it really does influence public confidence and trust.

Activity 8.6   *Decision making*

Consider the case study involving Peter Piper's letter to the Chief Executive of a Trust. Although we have no specific details in relation to the complaint, we do know that Peter was dissatisfied with the care that he received. We also know from Peter's letter that there is a lack of response to his complaint.

- From within the letter, identify three or four possible reasons why people complain about the NHS complaint handling process.

An outline answer is provided at the end of the chapter.

Peter states within his letter that if he does not receive an appropriate response to his complaint he will 'take the matter further'. The final step in the NHS complaints process is the *Parliamentary and Health Service Ombudsman* and this is where people generally go when the NHS has failed to address concerns. The Ombudsman aims to resolve complaints not only about the NHS, but Government departments and other public organisations.

The role of the Ombudsman is to:

*   listen to the human stories;
*   make judgements on complaints;
*   share insights from casework with others;
*   work alongside others to make public services better;
*   lead the way in making the complaints system better.

The Ombudsman makes reference to the fact that, when it comes to dealing with complaints handling and patient dissatisfaction, many hospitals are failing to respond well. The Ombudsman claims that Mid Staffordshire is not an isolated example. Around 10 per cent of all formal complaints about the health service seek a resolution from the Ombudsman.

Activity 8.7   *Reflection*

Think about your own practice experience to date.

*   Have you ever been in a situation where a patient, relative or carer has complained about healthcare?
*   Would you be able to support and signpost a patient, relative or carer who wanted to complain?
*   Do you know how to access the complaints policy within the Trust or organisation where you currently work?
*   Who actually deals with complaints handling within the Trust or organisation?

You might find it useful to discuss any thoughts or uncertainties with your practice mentor.

As this activity is for your own reflection, there is no answer at the end of the chapter.

It is important that we know how to handle complaints and appropriately support patients and relatives who feel that they want to complain. Complaints should not always be viewed as a failing in the service or the system, but as an opportunity to improve services and investigate systems that might have the potential to cause harm. It is vital that we measure patient experience in order for us to improve services and care delivery.

The Outcomes Framework – measuring patient experience

There are a number of national policy drivers that require Trusts and other healthcare organisations to measure and improve patient experience, including the provision of safe care. The NHS Outcomes Framework is one such driver. The main purpose of this framework is to provide a national overview as to how well the NHS is performing, and by acting as a catalyst to improve quality and encourage a change in culture and behaviour throughout the NHS.

The NHS Outcomes Framework reflects the vision set out in the White Paper, *Liberating the NHS* (DH, 2010c). The overall purpose is threefold:

* providing a national level overview of how well the NHS is performing;
* accounting for the effective spend of public money;
* acting as a catalyst for quality improvement throughout the NHS by encouraging a change in behaviour and culture. (Behaviour and culture are discussed more comprehensively in Chapter 9.)

Indicators in the NHS Outcomes Framework are grouped around five domains, which set out national outcomes that the NHS should be aiming to improve. Two domains are relevant to patient safety measurement and monitoring:

* **Domain 1**: Preventing people from dying prematurely;
* **Domain 5**: Treating and caring for people in a safe environment and protecting them from avoidable harm.

Commissioning for Quality and Innovation framework

The Commissioning for Quality and Innovation (CQUIN) framework is a system that was introduced in 2009 to make a proportion of the income that providers of healthcare receive conditional. In simple terms what this means is that people who provide healthcare need to demonstrate, on a yearly basis, that they are achieving quality improvement and innovation goals in specific areas of care. If goals are achieved, money is released. It is an incentive to improve patient safety in domains 1 and 5 of the NHS Outcomes Framework. Some goals are nationally determined, with others agreed locally. We now know that the NHS Outcomes Framework and policy direction need us to focus on a small number of key outcomes that we must measure together. The NHS Safety Thermometer is one such tool that has nationally determined goals that aim to deliver improvement at a local level.

NHS Safety Thermometer

The NHS Safety Thermometer (Qipp Safe Care Team, 2012) has been developed as an improvement tool, and to support the achievement of CQUIN through measuring, monitoring and analysing safe care. It is seen as a starting point for the development of a more sophisticated system of measurement. It also means that everyone is measuring the same information, in the same way, with the general aim of providing consistency.

The Safety Thermometer measures the proportion of patients who experienced four types of harm, compared to the proportion of patients who received harm-free care over a given period of time. More simplistically, the Safety Thermometer can be used to take the 'temperature' of your clinical setting, measuring baseline information about risk assessment, risk management and outcomes. The tool measures four high-volume patient safety issues that are tailored to the local clinical context:

- pressure ulcers;
- falls in care;
- urinary tract infection (patients who are in care with a urinary catheter);
- treatment for venous thromboembolism (VTE).

The patient safety issues highlighted are seen as 'nurse-sensitive' indicators. This means measuring the structure, processes and outcomes of nursing care. Not only are these issues viewed as complications of care, but they are also being referred to as harm that has been caused.

Activity 8.8   *Reflection and critical thinking*

Think about your current and previous practice placements. This might be in an acute Trust, the community, a care home, the private sector or another organisation that delivers care.

Consider the following questions.

- Is every nurse that you talk to aware of the NHS Safety Thermometer?
- Does every nurse know what the four high-volume patient safety issues are?
- Can you identify clinical settings that are actively collecting baseline information on any of the four identified issues? If so, how frequently is the data collected?
- Can you identify clinical settings that have changed approaches to care delivery as a direct result of the NHS Safety Thermometer?
- Can you think of any organisations or clinical settings where you have worked that display information publicly, in terms of the NHS Safety Thermometer?

A useful resource in relation to understanding the NHS Safety Thermometer is the '10 steps to success', which can be found at: http://harmfreecare.org/resources/nhsst-10steps

As this activity is for your own reflection and critical thinking, there is no answer at the end of the chapter.

It is recommended that every organisation must consider 'five things' if it wants to be successful in the implementation of the NHS Safety Thermometer:

1. SHARE
2. LEARN
3. MEASURE
4. ACTION
5. LEADERSHIP.

Activity 8.9   *Critical thinking*

- Consider the 'five things' every organisation must consider in order to be successful in the implementation of the NHS Safety Thermometer. What do you understand by each of those 'things' in terms of the Safety Thermometer? It might be useful to write your thoughts down on a piece of paper.

An outline answer is provided at the end of the chapter.

The national CQUIN goals are reviewed yearly and minor changes are made in light of current trends. This might influence the type of information or data we collect so that we can continue to improve care and patient safety in the four key areas identified.

National CQUIN goals for 2013/14

Four national CQUIN goals for 2013/14 have been highlighted. The two that are specific to safe care and link directly to the NHS Safety Thermometer are:

1. venous thromboembolism (VTE) and
   (a) that 95 per cent of the patient population are being risk assessed for VTE;
   (b) the achievement of a locally agreed goal, that all patients admitted with VTE are reviewed through root cause analysis (see pages 43–4 in Chapter 3);
2. the ability to demonstrate improvement against the NHS Safety Thermometer (excluding VTE), particularly in relation to pressure sores.

We have looked at national approaches to measuring safety and some of the policies that drive the safety agenda. Such measures can be tailored for use at a local level to meet the needs of organisations and clinical settings throughout the country. As patient safety is not only a national concern, we can look further and take into consideration internationally recognised approaches to measuring patient safety. Such approaches can be adapted and applied to our own Trusts and organisations.

Global Trigger Tool for Measuring Adverse Events

A relatively new method for measuring harm is known as the Global Trigger Tool for Measuring Adverse Events. One of the main aims is to enable a consistent and accurate measurement of harm. We know that traditional methods have focused on voluntary reporting and tracking errors. We appreciate that there are different approaches and inconsistencies in the ways in which we attempt to measure patient safety. More often than not errors, mistakes or mishaps in care delivery are not reported, unless the outcome had serious consequences for the patient, for example operating on the wrong body part or leaving instruments inside a patient.

Case study

Jean was admitted to hospital as an emergency for removal of her appendix. After her operation, surgeons realised that a swab was missing and that it had been left inside Jean.

They immediately carried out a second operation to remove the swab, but during this procedure a small part of a drain was left inside her abdomen. Jean was discharged from hospital three days later.

A few weeks passed, and Jean was taken back to hospital as she was seriously ill; she had developed a very high temperature and was in extreme pain.

Jean underwent a third operation to remove the drain fragment that had been left behind. As the drain was a 'foreign body', a large pus-filled abscess had developed within Jean's pelvis. The surgeons had no alternative but to form a colostomy and allow the damaged tissue time to heal. Jean will require further surgery to reverse the colostomy.

The Department of Health has categorised such incidents, as described in the case study involving Jean, as **never events**. This means they are incidents that are so serious they should never happen. In healthcare delivery there is an emphasis placed on 'never events' as these incidents are reported, but actually the picture is much greater, and the fact is that we have thousands of patient safety issues a year, many of which we know go unreported.

Jeremy Hunt, the Health Secretary, stated in 2013 that *the facts are clear – last year there were nearly half a million incidents that led to patients being harmed, and 3,000 people lost their lives while in the care of the NHS* (quoted by BBC News Health, 21 June); some of these incidents were categorised as 'never events'. The statistics presented may well be the 'tip of the iceberg', particularly when we know that many patient safety incidents are not reported. It is estimated that only 10 to 20 per cent of errors, mistakes and mishaps are reported. A more effective method is needed to measure adverse events so that improvements can be made.

We need to be able to measure safety more accurately and perhaps the Global Trigger Tool is a means of doing just that. It is a method for measuring the overall level of harm that may be occurring in a healthcare organisation. Trigger tools help to identify adverse effects and areas for improvement by regularly auditing a small sample of patient notes. Patient notes are reviewed to identify 'triggers' that might signal harm from patients' points of view. When a situation is identified that might have harmed a patient, teams are encouraged to take steps to improve the care process. Any change to the care process is monitored.

The tool provides instructions and forms for data collection that needs to track three measures:

1. the number of adverse events, or incidents, per 1,000 patient days;
2. the number of adverse events, or incidents, per 100 admissions;
3. the percentage of admissions with an adverse event, or incident.

The aim is to be able to track changes over time and demonstrate a reduction in monthly adverse events that have been identified.

Measuring safety culture

We have considered several different approaches to measuring patient safety but there is another measure that is worth thinking about and that is the measurement of safety culture. The current Health Secretary, Jeremy Hunt, believes that it is essential to *turn the tide* in relation to the levels of patients harmed in our care. Furthermore, he claimed that it is time *for a major rethink – a different kind of culture and leadership is required, where staff are supported to go with their instincts* (quoted by BBC News Health, 21 June 2013).

Manchester Patient Safety Framework

The Manchester Patient Safety Framework (MaPSaF) was introduced to healthcare in 2006 and is a tool that uses critical dimensions of patient safety to help teams assess their progress in developing a safety culture. The dimensions relate to areas where attitudes, values and behaviours about patient safety are likely to be reflected in the organisation's working practices. The tool has been developed to help healthcare teams and organisations reflect on their progress in developing a mature safety culture, supporting a drive towards cultural change.

Overall, a positive safety culture aims to create organisations that are open, just and informed, in which reporting and learning for errors, mistakes and mishaps are normal. It would appear that little has changed since MaPSaF was introduced in terms of safety culture and perhaps the time is right to revisit some of the key principles and themes outlined in the framework.

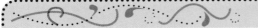

Chapter summary

It would appear that a key challenge remains in relation to measuring safety and that is the identification of a unified approach. The reality is that safety in relation to patient care delivery is very complex and we might need to rely on mixed approaches in terms of measuring patient safety. What is really worth noting is that information, measurements and data about the threats to patient safety can come from a variety of sources. They might be complementary to one another, but they are by no means the same. Each data information source or process has a unique perspective, with its own unique strengths and weaknesses. We need to recognise that there might be little or no overlap at all between each of these methods of measuring patient safety. Safety is sometimes viewed as the ability to anticipate and respond effectively to hazards and difficulties that we encounter when delivering care. Perhaps the more experienced we become within healthcare, the more able we are to deal with the constantly changing and hazardous healthcare environment. Measuring patient safety remains a global challenge and continues to be a priority for policy makers, healthcare providers, patients and the public.

Activities: brief outline answers

Activity 8.5: Critical thinking (page 138)

Some of the variables that might influence patients' satisfaction/dissatisfaction include age, gender, ethnicity, their presenting health issues, time that has elapsed since receiving the care, religious beliefs, engagement with the system/environment, perceptions of what constitutes 'good' care, previous care experiences, mental capacity, caring attitude, continuity of care, technical quality of care, accessibility and convenience, length of time between diagnosis and treatment, and pain management.

This list in not intended to be exhaustive and you might have identified additional or different variables.

Activity 8.6: Decision making (page 140)

In the case study you might have identified the following reasons:

*   a failure to understand the complaint and outcome sought by the complainant;
*   a failure to respond in writing to the complainant;
*   an inadequate apology;
*   no real acknowledgement of the mistake;
*   the verbal responses were not proportionate to the seriousness of the complaint.

Activity 8.9: Critical thinking (page 144)

The 'five things' every organisation must consider in order to be successful in the implementation of the NHS Safety Thermometer are:

1. SHARE
2. LEARN
3. MEASURE
4. ACTION
5. LEADERSHIP.

In terms of each 'thing' and how it applies to the Safety Thermometer you might have considered the following.

*   SHARE – This is about sharing good practice and ensuring that success is shared throughout the organisation in relation to care that is free from harm.
*   LEARN – By measuring all of your actions you will quickly be able to see what is working for your organisation. Some areas that are measured might be more successful than others. Acknowledge the less successful areas and move on, perhaps trying another approach that has been shared throughout the organisation.
*   MEASURE – Avoid measuring harm in isolation and consider looking at providing 'harm-free' care from a patient's perspective. Measurement is a way of recognising when something works well and it provides the necessary information in order to celebrate success and accomplishment within the team. It will enable the team to share good practice and service improvement throughout the wider organisation.
*   ACTION – This is about committing to specific actions, goal setting and working within a timeframe.
*   LEADERSHIP – Good strong leadership is paramount to success. Leadership is discussed more comprehensively in Chapter 9, but a motivated and driven day-to-day team leader who can engage with senior leaders is crucial to the success of delivery.

Further reading

Griffin, FA and Resar, RK (2009) *IHI Global Trigger Tool for Measuring Adverse Events*, 2nd edition. IHI Innovation Series White Paper. Cambridge, MA: Institute for Healthcare Improvement.

The authors of this White Paper state that tracking adverse events over time is a useful way to tell if any changes being made are improving the safety of care.

Parker, D, Lawrie, M, Carthey, J and Coultous, M (2008) The Manchester Patient Safety Framework: sharing the learning. *Clinical Risk*, 14(4): 140–2.

Useful websites

www.dh.gov.uk/en/publicationsandstatistics/Publications/PublicationsPolicyAnd Guidance/DH_122944

The NHS Outcomes Framework 2011/12 is available here.

www.dh.gov.uk/en/publicationsandstatistics/Publications/PublicationsPolicyAnd Guidance/DH_131700

The NHS Outcomes Framework 2012/13 is available here.

www.ihi.org/knowledge/Pages/Tools/IHIGlobalTriggerToolforMeasuringAEs.aspx

The Institute for Healthcare Improvement website describes how using triggers or clues to identify adverse events might be an effective method for measuring the overall level of harm in a healthcare organisation.

www.nrls.npsa.nhs.uk/resources/?entryid45=59796

The Manchester Patient Safety Framework (MaPSaF) is a tool to help NHS organisations and healthcare teams assess their progress in developing a safety culture. Comprehensive information in terms of the framework is provided here.

www.ombudsman.org.uk

Further information on the role and function of the Parliamentary and Health Service Ombudsman can be found at this website. The Ombudsman's principles and roles are clearly set out, signposting the public as to how to make a complaint. The main role is to investigate complaints, but the overall remit of the Ombudsman is far greater and considers influencing improvements in public services and informing public policy.

www.rcn.org.uk/_data/assets/pdf_file/0004/521833/17.13_Briefing_on_NHS_Complaints_ Review.pdf

Further information in relation to the review of complaints is available here.

Chapter 9
The influence of leadership and culture in managing patient safety

NMC Standards for Pre-registration Nursing Education

This chapter will address the following competencies:

Domain 1: Professional values

1. All nurses must practise with confidence according to *The Code: Standards of conduct, performance and ethics for nurses and midwives* (NMC, 2008), and within other recognised ethical and legal frameworks. They must be able to recognise and address ethical challenges relating to people's choices and decision making about their care, and act within the law to help them and their families and carers find acceptable solutions.

4. All nurses must work in partnership with service users, carers, families, groups, communities and organisations. They must manage risk, and promote health and well-being while aiming to empower choices that promote self-care and safety.

5. All nurses must fully understand the nurse's various roles, responsibilities and functions, and adapt their practice to meet the changing needs of people, groups, communities and populations.

7. All nurses must be responsible and accountable for keeping their knowledge and skills up to date through continuing professional development. They must aim to improve their performance and enhance safety and quality of care through evaluation, supervision and appraisal.

9. All nurses must appreciate the value of evidence in practice, be able to understand and appraise research, apply relevant theory and research findings to their work, and identify areas for further investigation.

Domain 4: Leadership, management and team working

1. All nurses must act as change agents and provide leadership through quality improvements and service development to enhance people's well-being and experiences of healthcare.

2. All nurses must systematically evaluate care and ensure that they and others use the findings to help improve people's experience and care outcomes and to shape future services.

6. All nurses must work independently as well as in teams. They must be able to take the lead in co-ordinating, delegating and supervising care safely, managing risk and remaining accountable for the care given.

NMC Essential Skills Clusters

This chapter will address the following ESCs:

Cluster: Care, compassion and communication

1. As partners in the care process, people can trust a newly registered graduate nurse to provide collaborative care based on the highest standards, knowledge and competence.

By entry to the register:

8. Demonstrates clinical confidence through sound knowledge, skills and understanding relevant to field.
9. Is self aware and self confident, knows own limitations and is able to take appropriate action.
10. Acts as a role model in promoting a professional image.

Cluster: Organisational aspects of care

14. People can trust the newly registered graduate nurse to be autonomous and confident as a member of the multi-disciplinary or multi-agency team and to inspire confidence in others.

By entry to the register:

8. Takes effective role within the team adopting a leadership role when appropriate.

15. People can trust the newly registered graduate nurse to safely delegate to others and to respond appropriately when a task is delegated to them.

By entry to the register:

2. Works within the requirements of *The Code* (NMC, 2008) in delegating care and when care is delegated to them.

16. People can trust the newly registered graduate nurse to safely lead, co-ordinate and manage care.

By entry to the register:

1. Inspires confidence and provides clear direction to others.
3. Bases decisions on evidence and uses experience to guide decision making.

17. People can trust the newly registered graduate nurse to work safely under pressure and maintain the safety of service users at all times.
18. People can trust the newly registered graduate nurse to enhance the safety of service users and identify and actively manage risk and uncertainty in relation to people, the environment, self and others.

By entry to the register:

9. Reflects on and learns from safety incidents as an autonomous individual and as a team member and contributes to team learning.
11. Assesses and implements measures to manage, reduce or remove risk that could be detrimental to people, self and others.
14. Works within policies to protect self and others in all care settings including the home care setting.

Chapter aims

After reading this chapter, you will be able to:

- identify how values and beliefs can influence the way in which we practise;
- explore situations where we accept and conform to organisational values and beliefs, rather than challenging them;
- recognise situations were leadership skills are required, specifically in relation to the safety of patients;
- understand how positive leadership can influence a safe working culture for both patients and staff.

Introduction

Scenario

Jason needs to attend a staff development day as part of his ongoing professional progress and the venue is 35 miles away from his current place of work. Jason realises that other people from the same Trust will need to attend. Transport links are limited and Jason knows that the venue has free car parking facilities. Jason suggests car sharing to four other members of staff who need to go. They willingly accept the offer, most of them stating, 'why didn't I think of that?' Jason had not realised that by suggesting they car share he was, in fact, taking on a leadership role.

The purpose of this chapter is to increase your awareness of how leaders and leadership can positively influence the patient safety culture. Beliefs and values will be considered alongside established behaviour and how such approaches to practice can influence organisational and safety culture. We will identify that the need for leadership skills is not confined to management roles. You will learn that any person providing assistance to others is acting as a leader. We will explore how the culture of an organisation is harder to measure than other aspects of performance and how safety culture can have both a positive and a negative impact on the care that we provide.

This chapter should be considered alongside *Leadership, Management and Team Working in Nursing* (Bach and Ellis, 2011), also in the Transforming Nursing Practice series, but the focus of this chapter will remain on how, as nurses and as leaders of care, we can influence the safety culture.

The influence of values and beliefs

Take some time to reflect on the personal values and beliefs that make you into the person you are. Also reflect on professional values and beliefs, and consider if they influence your behaviour.

- Do you act differently in your role as a nurse compared to when you are socialising with friends who perhaps don't understand the nature of your work?
- Does religion, family or the language you speak influence the way you behave?
- By behaving in the way you do as a nurse, or with your friends and family, what are you trying to achieve or gain?

As this activity is for your own reflection, there is no answer at the end of the chapter.

It is well accepted that our values and beliefs influence the way we live our lives. In very simplistic terms, values are ideas we hold to give meaning and significance to our lives and they underpin our beliefs. Beliefs influence the decisions we make, and the actions we take. Knowing the difference between values and beliefs can be confusing. We use both to guide us in the way that we act and behave.

Case study

Eleanor is 76 years old and has dementia. Eleanor has lived in a care home for many years after her husband John died. John was Eleanor's main carer and, although they have two children, neither of them was in a position to be able to provide the level of care that Eleanor needed to stay in her own home.

Over the last three months Eleanor has become increasingly frail. She has no visitors and her family only comes to see her at Christmas time. The family has not been involved in any 'do not attempt resuscitation' (DNAR) decisions.

Eleanor collapses on the way to the toilet. The nurse on duty has no option but to start resuscitation.

This case study demonstrates that, although our own values and beliefs might be to allow Eleanor to have a dignified death, professional values and beliefs differ. As there was no DNAR in place, attempts to resuscitate Eleanor needed to be made. Sometimes, as professionals, we can struggle with these types of decisions as they might not be what we would want to see happen to our own family or loved ones, going against our personal values and beliefs. Professional values and beliefs do influence the way in which we act, and the decisions we make in practice.

Case study

Daisy has recently been promoted to band 6 staff nurse on a very busy medical ward. She has worked on the ward since qualifying and over the last two years has developed her skills and knowledge base in relation to the patients she cares for. She is only a few months away from completing her degree programme, and although she has found some of the modules challenging she really feels that her approach to practice has improved. Daisy believes that all her hard work has been recognised by the fact that she was successful in securing the band 6 position. Daisy is confident that she is worthy and deserving of the post as she has always tried her very best, even though at times she has found it difficult to fit into the team.

As Daisy has been promoted, her band 5 post was advertised. Stephen, who has just completed his nursing degree, applied for the post and much to his own amazement was offered the job. Stephen didn't feel that he was the most appropriate candidate for the post, as he had never experienced a placement on a medical ward throughout his training. Stephen willingly accepted the post and, after having attending the Trust's induction and mandatory training programme, was keen to get started on the ward.

Daisy asked the senior sister if she could be Stephen's preceptor as this was now part of her new role. This was agreed. Daisy and Stephen worked well together, but Stephen felt intimidated by other members of the team when Daisy wasn't on duty.

Electronic prescribing had been introduced on to the ward six months before Stephen came into post. Stephen had some knowledge of the process from a previous placement but still lacked confidence in using the system. During drug rounds Stephen was frequently asked to write down the names of patients requiring injections and was told that, once all oral medication had been administered, they would come back to those patients requiring injections, using the paper as a guide. Stephen asked why he had been asked to do this. He was told that electronic prescribing had slowed drug rounds down and there wasn't the time to administer injections as well as oral medications. It was quicker and easier to do it this way. Stephen felt uncomfortable with this approach to medicines management but went along with the requests to administer injections in this way, as it seemed to have become a habit and accepted custom and practice on the ward. Stephen was desperate to fit into the ward team and didn't want to challenge those more senior to him. Although Daisy did not use this approach, every other member of the team did, and he knew that, because Daisy adhered to the Trust and Nursing and Midwifery Council (NMC) policies in relation to medicines management, she was unpopular.

When we consider the case study involving Daisy and Stephen it is important that we look at the bigger picture. We know that at times people deviate from policy, but the impact of this particular habit could have far-reaching consequences in relation not only to the safety of the patients on the ward, but to individuals within the organisation and the organisation itself. It is human nature to want to be accepted into a team, to feel a sense of belonging and acceptance. The case study clearly demonstrates that, in routine situations, such as a drug round, the team liked to work in a particular way. This could be viewed as established practice, work routine or an existing tradition that has developed over time; it has become part of the ward culture. Culture like this has been described as *how we do things around here* (Vincent, 2010, p271).

Activity 9.2 — *Reflection*

Aspects of the case study involving Daisy and Stephen might have parallels with your own practice experiences, where you have felt the need to conform to established practices and work routines, just to feel a sense of belonging.

Think back to a practice situation where you have felt the need to conform or comply. It could be in relation to manual handling, for example.

- Have you ever been asked to perform a manoeuvre that you know should not be used?
- How did this make you feel personally and professionally?
- Were you able to challenge the situation?
- Do you feel that you are more likely to conform and less likely to question practice with which you feel uncomfortable?
- Would you feel differently in a situation where a patient could be harmed?

Although this activity is for your own personal reflection, guidance and suggestions are given at the end of the chapter.

Sometimes it is very difficult to speak out when other professionals have values and beliefs that differ from your own, even if you observe working practices that are not as good as they should be, or practices that could result in causing harm to a patient.

Activity 9.3 — *Evidence-based practice and research*

- Why do nurses find it so difficult to speak out about poor practice?
- Are there implications or repercussions for those who do speak out?

An outline answer is provided at the end of the chapter.

Leadership and patient safety

Although we might find that certain situations go against our own personal and professional values and beliefs, it is in many cases easier to quietly allow an unsafe situation to continue, as it is much more difficult to speak up or intervene. Real leadership is displayed when you take action, or intervene in situations where the quality of patient care is at risk of being compromised. Sometimes it means challenging individuals more senior to yourself or those with more experience. Sometimes it means using your professional knowledge, skill and judgement to seek workable solutions and resolutions without causing conflict. Consider the following case study.

Case study

Patricia Batista has been assigned as your mentor throughout your eight-week community practice placement. Patricia is a very experienced staff nurse and has been qualified for 28 years. You believe Patricia to be a fantastic role model and mentor, with only one exception, and that is related to the technique she uses when administering subcutaneous Tinzaparin. Her technique is poor and you observe that there is an obvious gap between Patricia's theoretical knowledge base and current recommended best practice and local guidelines.

For three consecutive days you have watched Patricia administer subcutaneous Tinzaparin to Bill Forsyth using a poor technique. Bill was discharged from hospital after having a total hip replacement. You know that Bill will need to have subcutaneous Tinzaparin daily for four weeks after his surgery to prevent venous thromboembolism (VTE), as this is the recommended best practice. If Patricia continues to use such a poor technique when administering the injection, you know the therapeutic benefits will be greatly reduced and Bill could potentially suffer harm.

You consider that the quality of Bill's care is at risk of being compromised due to poor drug administration technique. You know that Bill is not receiving a therapeutic dose of Tinzaparin and, although he is not in any immediate danger, you worry that over time he is more likely to develop a VTE. This situation, if allowed to continue, could have a very serious outcome for Bill.

You recognise that the situation in relation to the way Patricia administers subcutaneous injections needs to change, and you know you have a professional and moral obligation to change this established practice. You are aware that this is a situation that you feel empowered to change, but you know that you lack the leadership skills that are necessary to deal with the situation effectively. Even though you do not have all the skills necessary to approach Patricia, you are also aware that harm could be unintentionally caused to Bill.

Activity 9.4   *Decision making*

Consider the case study involving Patricia.

- Would you feel able to take action in relation to Patricia's poor practice, or would you rather conform and allow the situation to continue?
- Do you feel that it would be within your remit to confront Patricia even though she is an experienced nurse?
- Would you feel able to approach this situation with Patricia? What strategies might you use?

Outline answers are provided at the end of the chapter.

Applying leadership skills, values and attitudes in practice is a key practical element of learning. Leadership should not be viewed as an optional role or function for nurses, and all nurses should have the necessary leadership skills to apply these in all aspects of their work. However, we do need to acknowledge that there may be a gap between educational preparation and complex practice settings, leaving nurses unprepared to provide effective frontline leadership.

The Report of the Mid Staffordshire NHS Foundation Trust Public Inquiry, released in February 2013, otherwise known as the Francis Report, highlights some of the challenges that leadership in nursing faces in an always demanding and ever changing NHS.

Key emerging themes in relation to nursing leadership

The Francis Report highlights key themes in relation to how the role of leader is universally recognised as being absolutely critical in the safe and effective care of patients. The report suggested wards that were well led generally provided acceptable standards of care. The terrible experiences endured by patients, relatives and carers came largely from wards that lacked strong, principled and caring leadership. One of several key leadership characteristics that all successful wards shared was that visible priority was given to the delivery of safe and excellent care of their patients. Francis (2013) also recognised that leadership is an essential ingredient of the work of every nurse and that more needs to be done to promote professional development in leadership within the profession.

Within our faculty of education, prior to students embarking on their final practice placement in year 3 (internship/guided option), we provide a leadership workshop across all fields of nursing. One of the activities of the leadership workshop is for students to consider three key questions in relation to leadership and how prepared they feel for their future working lives.

1. Do you see yourself as a leader of care?
2. Consider a positive mentor or role model in practice that you want to be like. What skills, qualities, values and attitudes does he or she have?
3. What skills, qualities, values and attitudes do you think a leader possesses? It might help to consider leaders you have observed in action, such as qualified staff who lead wards, units and teams.

Activity 9.5   *Reflection*

- Consider questions 1, 2 and 3 above. It might be interesting for you to ask other nursing students or colleagues in practice to work through the same activity and then compare your thoughts and feelings.

As questions 1 and 2 are for your own personal reflection, there is no answer at the end of the chapter. Some guidance and suggestions are provided in relation to question 3.

Hopefully, you will have found that Activity 9.5 has helped to reinforce that leadership skills are integral to the nursing role and that being exposed to skilled, positive leadership role modelling significantly enhances the learning experience.

Common themes that emerge when students within our faculty share their thoughts and feelings are that the vast majority of them, if not all, do not currently see themselves as leaders of care. We have already mentioned that people who offer guidance, support and care to patients or clients are classified as leaders. Students' responses to question 1 included the following:

'Not at present, I feel that I do not have the assertiveness skills to direct a team and I think this inability is due to a lack of confidence and belief in myself to be an effective nurse.'

'I don't see myself as a leader because I don't know if I can collate all my skills, knowledge and abilities together to be efficient, effective and a reliable patient advocate.'

'No, I think that I can project a good image on placement, but placements are too short to develop leadership skills.'

'I think that I can be a good leader with the right experience. I can lead my side of the ward and ask other staff to do certain jobs if needed, but a good leader is also a good team worker.'

'Currently I don't see myself as a leader but I know that I am able to "step up" to being one if and when I need to be. I feel awkward telling healthcare assistants and other staff members what needs to be done as they have perhaps been in their role for a while.'

'Not at the moment. In practice I find I have moments where a little leader part of me can come through, but as a general rule I feel I question myself too much. Past mentors, in fact most of them, have commented on my knowledge and ability, but I don't have the confidence in that. They've all pretty much said that I need to let go, stop over thinking and just go with it, because it's there. I think once I've qualified and my confidence and knowledge grows in the area I am working, I think the "leader" role may, hopefully, naturally follow.'

'Yes, I like to do my own thing, not necessarily follow other people. I like to lead people and get things organised.'

Key responses and words commonly associated with question 2 include the following:

knowledgeable, hard working, efficient, caring, compassionate, genuine, practices in the best interests of the patients, assertive, time to support staff team, resilience, taking an interest in patients, a sense of humour, respected by others, part of the team, those who are caring, organised and thorough, effective, good communication skills, firm but fair, good communication with staff, patients and relatives, experienced, kind, friendly, a good advocate, gives regular constructive feedback, professional, committed, empathetic, skilled, approachable, supportive, considerate, always cares for patients holistically, enjoys sharing their knowledge, the connection with patients on a real and very personal level, having a good working relationship with other members of staff, having a wide knowledge base on the areas of practice they work in, good listener.

You might have found similarities between your own thoughts and feelings and those of other student nurses. This activity might help you negotiate some personal and professional outcomes/proficiencies/competencies you would like to achieve during your next practice placement. It might be that you now have a better understanding as to how leadership applies to your own professional practice.

So how can leaders influence a safety culture?

Leadership continues to be one of the most written-about and studied topics and it is important to recognise that leadership opportunities are available throughout our lives and professional work. They are not simply the point at which we finish a course of study or achieve a particular level of certification. Leadership is not confined to those in management roles and it is worth highlighting that any person who provides assistance to others is demonstrating leadership skills. As emphasised by the Francis Report, leadership skills are integral to the nursing role; a student nurse is a leader to patients and clients.

The Royal College of Nursing (RCN), in collaboration with the Department of Health, the NMC and patient and service organisations, developed the *Principles of Nursing Practice*. The *Principles*, launched by the RCN in November 2010, describe what everyone can expect from nursing. The eighth, Principle H, is concerned with leadership and states, *Nurses and nursing staff lead by example, develop themselves and other staff, and influence the way care is given in a manner that is open and responds to individuals needs.*

Activity 9.6 — *Reflection*

- Think about what leadership means to you. Can you recall a situation where you have acted in the role of a leader? It may well have been a situation when you were at school or during an out-of-school activity. Write down 20 words you would associate with the role of a leader. You might want to discuss this with a peer or your mentor. Write down the name you are called or known by, and for each initial try and think of a word that is usually associated with leadership and reflects your personality, for example:
  Sensitive
  Trusting
  Empowering
  Passionate
  Humble
  Assertive
  Nurturing
  Inspirational
  Enthusiastic.
- Find a job description for a junior staff nurse from your current place of work or use an online resource, and look to see how frequently words associated with leadership are used to define the role.
- If you had to choose just five key words to describe a leader or leadership, which five would you select?
- How many of the words you have chosen reflect common themes or words used in Activity 9.5, question 2? Do good mentors and positive role models demonstrate positive leadership traits?

No answer is given in relation to personal reflection, but some words that are associated with the role of a leader, or leadership, can be found at the end of the chapter.

We have now established that strong, caring and positive leadership can influence a safe and effective care experience for patients and clients. Wong and Cummings (2007) write about how positive leadership increased patient satisfaction and reduced the number of adverse incidents. Furthermore, provision of high-quality nursing care, together with the nurturing of a culture of innovation and support, is very much reliant on effective leadership skills.

Leadership and organisational culture are said to be very tightly intertwined. Leadership has been proposed as a key latent factor influencing the safety culture of an organisation, the likelihood of errors occurring and the way in which these are managed. The development of a positive safety culture should be within the context of the organisational culture as a whole and not viewed as a separate entity.

Defining culture

The word 'culture' has many different meanings.

Activity 9.7   *Reflection*

- People view the term 'culture' in different ways, so try to identify different types of culture. What does the word 'culture' mean to you?
- Try to define or describe organisational culture. It might be useful to write your definition or description down.

Outline answers are provided at the end of the chapter.

Organisational culture would seem to refer to the beliefs and values that have existed within the system for a long time; going back to the statement made earlier it could be described as 'how we do things around here'. Organisational culture has been described as the shared values, beliefs or perceptions held by employees within an organisation or an organisational unit (Robbins and Coulter, 2005).

Case study

As part of your personal and professional development you have been given the opportunity to attend the next Executive Board Meeting. This is an informal meeting of the Board, but nonetheless you appreciate how important such meetings are. You want to create a good impression and you want to present yourself in a professional and appropriate manner. You have spent some time ensuring that your uniform is clean and worn correctly, your shoes are polished and your hair is neat and tidy. By doing this you feel that you are upholding the values, beliefs and perceptions of the nursing profession and the Trust.

You arrive at the meeting venue in good time. When you open the door of the boardroom you find that it is not at all what you expected. The lighting is soft, and classical music is playing gently in the background. There is a wall mural of a beach and palm trees. The secretary greets you warmly, but you are so shocked to see her wearing a grass skirt and flip-flops.

The circumstances in the case study might seem extreme, but we can become complacent about organisation culture. If you had walked into the boardroom where the secretary wore a suit and the atmosphere was closer to that of a traditional business environment, you would not have given the circumstances a second thought. The scenario depicted an organisational culture that was very different from your expectations. It feels strange.

People are quick to recognise organisational cultures that are different from their own; they are usually so immersed in their own cultures that they take them for granted and sometimes have a hard time acknowledging they actually exist. The problem with becoming so immersed in the organisational culture is that poor practice and negative behaviours go unnoticed. What was once unacceptable is now an accepted tradition.

Francis (2013) recommends that an understanding of existing culture needs to be found so that the unacceptable behaviours can be identified and avoided in the future.

The culture within an organisation is very important, playing a large role in whether it is a happy and healthy environment in which to work. When the interaction between the leadership and employees is good, this will make a significant contribution to team communication and collaboration, enhancing job satisfaction (Tsai, 2011).

A theme that runs throughout the Francis Report (2013) is that of values in relation to culture. If we now consider culture in terms of beliefs, values and professional standards, what the Francis Report suggests is that a consistent culture produces the best chance for all patients to be treated in accordance with acceptable fundamental standards of safety and quality. That would require the NHS and all who work in it to develop and adhere to a common set of standards and values.

Case study

Bill has worked in the maintenance department of a large NHS Trust for several years. He has seen many changes and been part of two major restructuring processes. Bill's work request sheet for the day requires him to attend ward 18 to repair a faulty lock on the bathroom door and replace a cracked windowpane.

Bill arrives on the ward. He senses that the ward is very busy; staff don't have time to direct him to the cracked windowpane. Bill decides that the best approach would be to attend to the faulty bathroom lock first; at least he knows where the bathroom is. He sets about replacing the lock. While he is in the bathroom he can hear faint cries from the nearby toilet – 'Hello, is anybody there?' Bill carries on with his task. He wants to go and see if he can assist the patient in the toilet but he knows that it is not in his remit to do so. Bill tries to catch someone's attention but everyone is so busy. He leaves the ward, and the patient.

At first glance, Bill's approach within the case study might not seem that unreasonable. Bill would have offered the patient assistance if he had followed his own values and beliefs, but the organisational culture dictated that it was not in Bill's remit to offer assistance to the patient. However, the patient might have come to harm as a result of Bill not acting on his own values and beliefs.

If we now consider this case study in the context of 'the NHS and all who work in it should develop and adhere to a common set of standards and values', Bill might have felt more empowered to provide some form of assistance to the patient.

Francis (2013) makes reference to the fact that staff such as Bill are just as much part of the team working for the patients' benefit as are the nursing and medical staff. All staff need to be made part of an overall NHS culture. A shared common culture needs a commitment to shared common values. The challenge that the NHS now faces is how to achieve this.

A safety culture

Leadership needs to be recognised as a key influence of an organisation's safety culture. If we consider culture in the context of providing healthcare and, even more specifically, organisational safety, the concept becomes very difficult to actually define and definitely more difficult to measure in terms of patient safety.

By taking overall culture in healthcare just one step further, the Francis Report hoped that a safety culture would be an inherent component: *A culture which aspires to cause no harm and to provide adequate, and, where possible, excellent care and treatment might be called a 'safety culture'* (Francis, 2013, vol. 3, p1359).

Activity 9.8   *Critical thinking*

There are many definitions for 'safety culture'; not all are associated with the provision of healthcare.

- Write down on a piece of paper key words or phrases that you think might go towards the definition of a 'safety culture'.
- Try to find a definition that you feel would be appropriate to apply to the NHS.

As this activity involves your own critical thinking, there is no answer at the end of the chapter.

Although it would seem that there are many definitions in relation to what a safety culture actually is, a common theme emerges and that is about having a shared set of safety values and beliefs. The Advisory Committee on the Safety of Nuclear Installations (ACSNI) in 1993 developed one particular definition that is still widely used today:

> *The safety culture of an organisation is the product of individual and group values, attitudes and perceptions, competencies and patterns of behaviour that determine the commitment to, and the style and proficiency of, an organisation's health and safety.*

Subcultures

It is important to note that we can often view safety through subcultures, rather than sharing an overall view of safety as suggested by the definition offered. Francis (2013) also suggests that the NHS needs to strive towards a shared common culture that has a set of shared common values. We have discussed through the case study involving Daisy and Stephen (see page 153) that within an organisation there are often different groups of staff who have their own values and beliefs, resulting in their own 'way of doing things'. They might have different levels of concern for safety issues; in effect, they have their own safety subculture. Subcultures within an organisation can lead to misunderstanding or conflict between groups, but this is not always viewed negatively as different perspectives and a diversity of views can have a positive influence on safety. This allows people to raise concerns and voice opinions, and it might be one way of bringing subcultures together in order to share understanding in relation to situations that have caused harm to patients. The presence of subcultures within a large organisation such as the NHS might suggest that it would be very difficult to achieve a common safety culture.

Glendon and McKenna (1995) claim that organisations with a positive safety culture have effective communication strategies. Once again, this is based on communication that considers shared beliefs and values in relation to the importance of safety. Confidence in effective preventative measures is also considered to be an important factor in creating a positive safety culture. Leadership walk rounds are perhaps just one way of achieving this.

Leadership walk rounds

Leadership walk rounds are one example where safety culture and leadership are explicitly linked; they provide an informal method for leaders to talk with frontline staff about safety issues in the organisation and show their support for reporting errors. In order for walk rounds to be successful a great deal of organisational will is required. The aim of leadership walk rounds is to implement a patient safety culture that bridges the gap between leaders and frontline staff. Value can be added to the patient safety agenda through leadership walk rounds by breaking down barriers between leaders and frontline staff, opening channels of communication in relation to identifying situations that may cause harm, and gathering information to enhance decision making around patient safety. Leadership walk rounds need to be considered in the context of the organisation's readiness to provide time and support to leaders, organisational resources and patient safety priorities. Once in place it is important to consider how to sustain motivation and allocate resources appropriately to allow walk rounds to become embedded within the safety culture of the organisation. Walk rounds would seem to be an effective method for engaging leadership, identifying safety issues and supporting a culture of safety using a non-threatening approach for those who provide frontline care. Focusing solely on safety during these rounds has been recognised as a successful strategy for promoting and creating a safety culture, rather than discussing other areas of concern, for example staffing levels. Leadership walk rounds can develop a stronger and more unified safety culture.

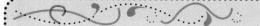

Chapter summary

This chapter has considered how professional values and beliefs can influence the way in which we practise and how in certain situations it is sometimes easier to conform than challenge established traditions or customs. We have noted that those who provide advice, support, care and guidance are leaders and that good leadership and role modelling is linked to a positive safety and organisational culture. We know that traditionally healthcare has had a culture of blame, where people are often punished for making errors. The patient safety agenda strives to create a culture of safety where frontline staff are comfortable speaking up about errors and situations that have caused harm, and leadership walk rounds are one method whereby we can encourage this dialogue to take place.

Activities: brief outline answers

Activity 9.2: Reflection (page 154)

It is not uncommon to want to feel part of a team and to fit in. It is well recognised within nursing that there are times when compliance and/or conformity seems like the only option. Over time and with experience come confidence, knowledge and the ability to be more assertive and to speak up. Nursing culture does exist but nurses do need to be empowered to speak out against poor practice or practice that may harm a patient.

Activity 9.3: Evidence-based practice and research (page 154)

Reporting poor practice is a moral and professional obligation. Nurses find it difficult to speak out about poor practice for several reasons, including:

- a fear of being marginalised or silenced;
- powerlessness;
- frustration;
- fear of disciplinary action.

Implications or repercussions for those who do speak out can be either personal or professional, including:

- personal attacks that may come from colleagues and the organisation;
- insomnia, headaches and fatigue;
- animosity and resentment that can be so great there is no other choice than to leave the organisation;
- punitive transfer to another clinical environment.

Activity 9.4: Decision making (page 155)

As nurses we would have a professional obligation to approach Patricia, regardless of how experienced we are, if we believe that she lacks competence in relation to a skill, in this case subcutaneous injection technique.

A student nurse is a leader to patients and clients. Tackling poor practice or a lack of competence is everyone's responsibility. As there is potential within the case study for Bill to develop a VTE, the student should feel able to approach Patricia. The student should be able to recognise that Patricia needs to be providing a high standard of practice and care at all times, making the care of people her first concern.

There are various ways to tackle poor practice or lack of competence. The easiest way, as in the case study involving Patricia, would be to ask her directly why she administers subcutaneous injections in the way she does. If Patricia is defensive, or she is unable to answer your question, return to the evidence base, as there may be a rationale or another useful explanation. If you are certain that the practice is poor, you may feel that you can present the evidence base in a non-threatening manner. Explain to Patricia the most up-to-date evidence base, and offer to demonstrate subcutaneous injection technique if you feel confident to do so. Local policy/guidelines might provide an opportunity to discuss poor practice or, in Patricia's case, a lack of competence. If you feel that Patricia cannot accept her practice is poor or that she lacks the competence, it would be appropriate to take the situation further. This is when it can become more challenging, as you would need to address the situation with a more senior member of the team, or alternatively Patricia's line manager. Finally, if the situation was allowed to continue and the patient was potentially at risk, an incident report should be completed so that further action can be taken. A useful online document is available from the NMC, which offers guidance and support in relation to raising concerns. This can be found at www.nmc-uk.org/raisingconcerns.

Activity 9.5: Reflection (page 156)

In thinking about question 3, by considering other activities within the chapter you will know that attitudes, beliefs and values shape behaviour. There are several forms of leadership, including situational, transformational, charismatic, authentic, distributed, transactional and servant/team. To gain a better understanding of leadership and its different forms, it would be beneficial to read *Leadership, Management and Team Working in Nursing* (Bach and Ellis, 2011). Regardless of the form, key values that you might have identified include honesty, communication, discipline, responsibility, trust, level-headedness, fairness, courage, vision, wisdom, passion, intelligence, humility, strategic thinking, integrity, persistence, among others.

Activity 9.6: Reflection (page 158)

Words frequently associated with leaders or leadership include purpose, integrity, values, strategy, principles, humility, passion, delegation, empowerment, sincerity, risk, confidence, commitment, wisdom, people, honesty, compassion, sensitivity, determination, courage, loyalty, patience, fairness, management, control, supervision, inspire, mentor, purpose, communicate, competence, commitment, organiser, visionary, diplomatic, transparency, commanding, adaptable, trustworthy, strategic, principled, passionate, humble, wise, courageous, vulnerable, focused, curious, trusting, consistency and teamwork.

This list is by no means exhaustive.

Activity 9.7: Reflection (page 159)

Culture can be viewed as the customs, arts and social interactions of a particular nation, people or other social group. Culture can also be viewed as an appreciation of art and human intellectual achievement (appreciation of classical music, going to the ballet, enjoying gourmet food). The attitudes, feelings and ideas you perceive on a day-to-day basis are all examples of culture.

Further reading

Bach, S and Ellis, P (2011) *Leadership, Management and Team Working in Nursing.* Exeter: Learning Matters.

This book is part of the Transforming Nursing Practice series and discusses comprehensively the concepts of leadership and management in nursing. This book is extremely useful to anyone working in health or social care who has an element of leadership and management in his or her role.

Levett-Jones, T and Lathlean, J (2009) 'Don't rock the boat': Nursing students' experiences of conformity and compliance. *Nurse Education Today*, 29(3): 342–9.

If you want to read more about conformity and compliance, try this particular article, which is based on students' experiences in relation to 'fitting in' to clinical practice and placements.

Temple, J (2012) *Becoming a Registered Nurse*. Exeter: Sage/Learning Matters.

Chapter 4 of this book is useful in providing additional scenarios in relation to your role as a leader and how this can influence and impact on other staff. Emotional intelligence in leadership, which can be found on page 66, is particularly useful in the context of culture and organisational goals.

Useful websites

www.gov.uk/government/uploads/systems/uploads/attachment_data/file/dh_125985.pdf

This Department of Health document is the Government's response to the recommendations in *Frontline Care: The report of the Prime Minister's Commission on the Future of Nursing and Midwifery in England*. This is a useful read, particularly for those preparing for interview or role transition.

www.midstaffspublicinquiry.com/report

The final Francis Report of 2013 can be found here. The executive summary and volumes 1, 2 and 3 can be viewed online. Podcasts and downloads are also available to view. Anyone involved with delivering healthcare and particularly those applying for jobs would be advised to read at least the executive summary and recommendations.

www.nmc-uk.org/Documents/NMC-Publications/238747_NMC_Standards_for_medicines_management.pdf

At this web page, remind yourself about *Standards for Medicines Management*.

www.nmc-uk.org/Publications/Standards/The-code/Introduction

And at this web page, remind yourself about *The Code: Standards of conduct, performance and ethics for nurses and midwives*.

www.rcn.org.uk/development/practice/principles

The *Principles of Nursing Practice*, launched by the RCN in November 2010, can be found here.

Chapter 10
Patient safety – what next?

continued . . . •••

By entry to the register:

9. Acts as an effective role model in decision making, taking action and supporting others.

Chapter aims

After reading this chapter, you will be able to:

* consolidate the concepts of patient safety and risk;
* glean an understanding of the political drivers in safety improvement;
* consider your own personal and professional development needs in relation to promoting safety.

Introduction

Scenario

At a recent tutorial with a nursing student, the lecturer was discussing the recommendations in the report of the Mid Staffordshire NHS Foundation Trust Public Inquiry (Francis, 2013). She was reinforcing the importance of risk managing situations, recording and reporting, and raising concerns. The student nodded but commented: 'You and I aren't going to change the world, though, are we?'

In the final chapter of our journey, it seems prudent to conclude by exploring the way forward in patient safety and managing risk. We will start by acknowledging the complexities of addressing patient safety and risk initiatives in an ever changing health service. We will then focus on the recommendations in the Francis Report, mentioned above, because it is a very timely and pivotal report that will undoubtedly have a profound effect on the health service and in particular on nursing. We will then go on to examine our own responsibilities in maintaining patient safety and summarise the skills set required of us to do so effectively.

We will refer to a variety of activities and strategies that are currently being utilised in clinical settings to promote patient safety. Finally, after reading the chapter, students and registrants should have a clear knowledge of what is expected of them in the promotion of patient safety and risk management. We may not be able to change the world, but each contribution, however small, could undoubtedly contribute to a culture of safety.

This book has focused on 'things going wrong' in healthcare delivery. We must remind ourselves, of course, that things do go right most of the time and that the standards of healthcare delivery and nursing care in the UK are excellent in many areas.

The changing infrastructure of the NHS

We have looked at the frameworks and models within the NHS that facilitate the promotion of patient safety. We know that nurses and others have a responsibility to contribute to safety in an ever changing healthcare arena. Readers of this book may be left a little daunted about what exactly is the requirement to report incidents and to whom. The NHS is victim to many infrastructure changes influenced by political and social policies. For example, the NPSA has been abolished in its original form and its functions distributed elsewhere. No doubt, by the time this book is published there will have been numerous other departmental changes. New initiatives will eventually replace CQUIN, the Safety Thermometer and other tools. This can present a problem to healthcare professionals, who can often become confused and feel that it is difficult to keep up with changes and keep abreast of policy. Change is, however, inevitable in healthcare services and something all of us have to embrace. Better effective communication systems should facilitate this and help with the dissemination of information to staff. Nurses are required to maintain current and evidence-based practice and we recommend that you need to sustain a sense of political awareness also.

The influence of the Francis Report

The authors have chosen to focus on the recommendations in the final report of the Mid Staffordshire NHS Foundation Trust Public Inquiry (Francis, 2013) to shape this chapter, as it will undoubtedly be an important driver for improving patient safety. It was published in February 2013 following the earlier report published in 2010. It focused on the shortcomings of a hospital that failed hundreds of patients and put corporate interests ahead of patient safety. The patients were failed by a system that ignored warning signs. The executive summary as well as the complete report can be accessed at www.midstaffspublicenquiry.com.

The report was published at the time of writing this chapter and so it is therefore timely when examining the way forward in patient safety. Interestingly, the report reinforces much of what we have written about in the preceding chapters, but it has been followed by much discussion and debate about how best to implement these recommendations in healthcare organisations while acknowledging the complexities.

The recommendations

The report made 290 recommendations designed to change the institutional culture that exists in many healthcare organisations and make sure that patients come first. The recommendations are centred around promoting a culture that is patient centred, intolerance of non-compliance with fundamental standards, openness and transparency, candour to patients, strong cultural leadership and caring, compassionate nursing, and useful and accurate information and services.

Below is a small selection of the recommendations that we have picked out as being particularly relevant to your practice as a student or registrant in relation to patient safety.

Francis Report recommendations

Putting the patient first

Recommendation no. 5

In reaching out to patients, consideration should be given to including expectations in the NHS Constitution that:

- staff put patients before themselves;
- they will do everything in their power to protect patients from harm;
- they will be honest and open with patients regardless of the consequences for themselves;
- where they are unable to provide the assistance a patient needs, they will direct them where possible to those who can do so;
- they will apply the NHS values in all their work.

Fundamental standards of behaviour

Recommendation no. 11

- Healthcare professionals should be prepared to contribute to the development of, and comply with, standard procedures in the areas in which they work. Their managers need to ensure that their employees comply with these requirements. Staff members affected by professional disagreements about procedures must be required to take the necessary corrective action, working with their medical or nursing director or line manager within the Trust, with external support where necessary. Professional bodies should work on devising evidence-based standard procedures for as many interventions and pathways as possible.

Recommendation no. 12

- Reporting incidents of concern relevant to patient safety, compliance with fundamental standards or some higher requirement of the employer needs to be not only encouraged but insisted upon. Staff are entitled to receive feedback in relation to any report they make, including information about any action taken or reasons for not acting.

Caring for the elderly

Recommendation no. 240

- Hygiene: All staff and visitors need to be reminded to comply with hygiene requirements. Any members of staff, however junior, should be encouraged to remind anyone, however senior, of these.

Recommendation no. 241

- Provision of food and drink: The arrangements and best practice for providing food and drink to elderly patients require constant review, monitoring and implementation.

Recommendation no. 242

- Medicines administration: In the absence of automatic checking and prompting, the process of the administration of medication needs to be overseen by the nurse in charge of the ward, or his/her nominated delegate. A frequent check needs to be done to ensure that all patients have received what they have been prescribed and what they need. This is particularly the case when patients are moved from one ward to another, or they are returned to the ward after treatment.

Recommendation no. 243

- Recording of routine observations: The recording of routine observations on the ward should, where possible, be done automatically as they are taken, with the results being immediately accessible to all staff electronically in a form enabling progress to be monitored and interpreted. If this cannot be done, there needs to be a system whereby ward leaders and named nurses are responsible for ensuring that the observations are carried out and recorded.

Activity 10.1   *Critical thinking*

Think about your own healthcare Trust where you have been working on placement.

- How do you think it is addressing the above to make sure standards are met?
- Do you think the recommendations are achievable?

As this activity is based on your own experience, there is no answer at the end of the chapter.

Many of the recommendations need to be embraced by Trust Boards in healthcare organisations if they are to be effective, but it is up to all of us to 'do our bit' in ensuring that patient safety comes first. The Trust in the Mid Staffordshire case was criticised for putting its targets first before safety; it did not listen to those who raised concerns; there was a culture of 'bullying' and intimidation when staff did attempt to draw attention to concerns; and patient stories went unheard. In Chapters 5 and 6 we explored the concept of raising concerns and many of you reading this book and the Francis Report will no doubt reflect on the potential negative consequences that are associated with whistleblowing for the individual, which could be you!

> **Case study**
>
> *Sharon is a ward sister on the stroke rehabilitation unit of a large district hospital. She is new in post and is keen to build a good team who deliver excellent care and she hopes to promote a just and safe culture within her ward environment. Sharon has a good rapport with her team. She demonstrates a transformational leadership style and is generally well respected. It has come to her attention that three medicines administration errors have been made during a period of two weeks by two different registrants. None of the incidents led to patient harm and they were reported using the incident reporting system. Sharon was concerned about the incidents and felt strongly that she needed to take steps to avoid them occurring in the future. She had already investigated and interviewed the staff involved privately. She felt that the nurses had not acted unprofessionally but that they had made genuine mistakes. She decided that the best way to approach the issue and attempt to improve safety on medicine rounds was to discuss the incidents at the two-weekly ward meeting. She would not identify any staff involved but instead she would discuss the incidents and encourage the team to think of ways in which future incidents could be avoided.*

This case study is an example of a ward manager adopting an open approach in dealing with what could have potentially led to poor practice and entrenched behaviour. Instead she decided to utilise the opportunity to involve the team in seeking a solution. By taking this open and transparent approach Sharon is probably more likely to foster a culture of honesty and openness in her team.

> **Activity 10.2**   *Reflection*
>
> • With a fellow student or colleague, discuss some reasons why nurses may not raise a concern about practice.
>
> *An outline answer is provided at the end of the chapter.*

There may be a variety of reasons that may prevent you from speaking out, but by doing so you may help to improve the patient experience. As a student or newly qualified nurse you may consider yourself to be the 'junior member of the firm', but remember we are bound by our professional *Code* and have a duty to speak up.

Are nurses protected against speaking out?

There are well-documented reports of nurses being discouraged from speaking out. However, in order to promote a more transparent, enabling culture, the term 'whistleblowing' has largely been replaced by 'raising concerns'. 'Whistleblowing' is a term that has been associated with negativity and the fear of recourse. We have to remember, though, that by speaking out some nurses have managed to instigate changes that have improved patient care and safety. We have already discussed raising concerns in Chapters 5 and 6. There is evidence that an increasing number of healthcare providers are working hard to develop a culture that is open, transparent and candid. The Public Interest Disclosure Act 1998 was introduced to provide protection for those who honestly raise genuine concerns about wrongdoing or workplace malpractice. Provided that they are acting in the public interest and not for personal gain, if they are dismissed or victimised this Act provides workers with protection when raising concerns internally. Protection is also available for disclosures to regulatory bodies and, in exceptional circumstances, wider disclosures to external bodies such as the media. The NMC (2010b) advises its members to consult its guidance on raising and escalating concerns before following this route.

Scenario

You are a newly qualified registered nurse working on a ward with predominantly elderly patients, some of whom are confused. You notice that an elderly gentleman in the side ward is trying to attract someone's attention and he appears agitated. Just as you are about to attend to him two call bells sound simultaneously. The late shift has gone off for a meal break so there are three staff left on the ward, which is usual practice: yourself, another registrant and a healthcare assistant. A visitor then runs to you and informs you that her mother is desperate for a bedpan. One of your colleagues has gone on an errand to X-ray and the other colleague is at the other end of the ward attending to a distressed patient.

The scenario above is not unusual and many of you may have been in a similar situation. You need to prioritise what needs to be done, but whatever decision you make it is likely that patients will have to wait for attention. To the individual patient and their relatives this can seem frustrating and some may consider their wait as an example of substandard care. In the short term, you may be able to handle the situation and avert dissatisfaction by good communication and interpersonal skills. In the longer term, you could discuss the situation with your line manager so that prioritisation and organisation of work may help to prevent a similar situation from occurring again. It may have been possible to stagger meal breaks, allowing more staff cover. The errand to X-ray could perhaps have been postponed to a more suitable time, resulting in more staff presence on the ward. Maybe there is a business case for reviewing staff numbers and skill mix. On the other hand, it might not be possible to make these changes.

The scenario above is multi-faceted and complex, but there are other situations where solutions may seem more straightforward.

Activity 10.3   *Critical thinking*

Imagine you are working in the critical care department as a student nurse. The infection control policy is well established and all staff are required to wash their hands between attending to patients. You observe that Dr Bull, the consultant anaesthetist, never washes his hands between patients. Most of the staff apart from the ward sister prefer to ignore this as he is not the most approachable person. He can be quite intimidating and he is seen as a senior figure in this department.

- Would you feel comfortable raising concerns in this situation? If so, then how? Explain your approach.

An outline answer is provided at the end of the chapter.

Despite the dilution of paternal hierarchies in nursing and healthcare, hierarchies do still exist. While many nurses would feel confident to approach a senior figurehead and remind him of the importance of hand washing and adhering to policy, there are many who would not feel they could approach the individual, but as the Francis Report (2013) recommends, it is everyone's responsibility no matter how junior.

Nursing and healthcare are currently in the media spotlight. The previous chapters have explored why and considered the potential impact this can have on patients and relatives. We have seen how patient safety and risk management has evolved over past centuries and decades, but have we really moved on from Florence Nightingale's declaration that *hospitals should do the sick no harm*?

In her *Notes on Nursing* (1860/1969), she put forward her ideas on hygiene, the deteriorating patient, nutrition, hydration and compassion. She based her observations on mortality rates, just as the Mid Staffordshire Inquiry did. They were written over 100 years ago and health-care knowledge has advanced considerably, yet to read some of the issues raised in the reports discussed in this book it would appear to some that we have made little progress in terms of care.

The role of risk assessment tools in patient safety

We have already discussed risk assessment and risk management in previous chapters. There is no doubt that managing risk is crucial. However, it should be remembered that the use of risk assessment tools is no substitute for clinical decision making and professional judgement. Rather, risk assessment tools should be used as an adjunct to help the nurse formulate a plan of care.

> ## Activity 10.4   *Reflection*
>
> - Make a list of examples of risk assessment tools you have used in clinical practice and discuss with a peer or colleague whether you feel they have been useful in helping you determine a patient's needs.
>
> *An outline answer is provided at the end of the chapter.*

Remember that risk assessments should be carried out by staff who are trained to use the various tools required. They should also possess the level of expertise required to make a sound clinical judgement using the best evidence available.

Documentation and record keeping

Although we have discussed the importance of incident reporting and reporting concerns throughout the book, it is perhaps prudent to remind the reader of the importance of record-keeping skills. Although nurse education and practice providers emphasise the importance of documentation, it is alarming how many nurses and healthcare professionals find themselves at fitness to practise hearings as a result of poor record keeping. Record keeping is fundamental to healthcare delivery. The healthcare professional has both a legal and professional obligation to maintain clear and accurate records. Any form of recorded patient information should stand up to legal scrutiny, including incident reports. Many professionals therefore have concerns as to whether their records will stand up to legal and professional scrutiny. The NMC (2009) provides guidelines on standards for record keeping (due for review in October 2013) and the reader is advised to access the guidelines, which set out good practice. In addition, most healthcare providers will have developed policies in relation to record keeping practice and you are advised to read your local placement policy. A good standard of record keeping is the sign of a safe practitioner and helps to protect the welfare of patients. Good records promote high standards of care, continuity of care, better communication and an accurate account of treatment and care delivery (Lynch, 2009).

Skills essential to promoting patient safety

So what have we learned about the skills we need to protect patients from harm?

> ## Activity 10.5   *Critical thinking*
>
> - Write down a summary of the skills you now think you need to develop as a nurse to promote patient safety and prevent harm, based on the preceding chapters and your own experiences.
>
> *An outline answer is provided at the end of the chapter.*

As you develop your knowledge and skills, you will be aware of your own learning needs and areas you need to develop. This will vary from individual to individual and your education supervisors as well as practice mentors will help you to identify such areas.

Building a wall of confidence

Within our faculty of education, at the end of a first-year nursing module delivered to all fields of nursing, we provide a workshop, one of the aims of which is to allow students to 'build a wall of confidence'. The wall of confidence is based on their philosophical beliefs about nursing and 'putting the patient first'. It is also about restoring patients' trust in the health service and promoting a safe environment. Figure 10.1 shows some of the ideas posted on the wall of confidence.

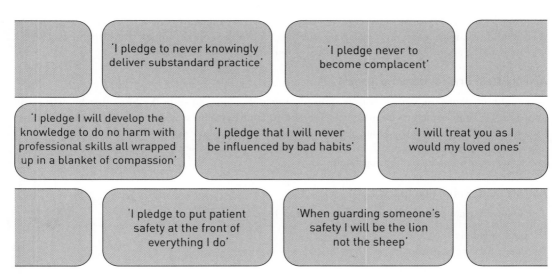

'I pledge to never knowingly deliver substandard practice'

'I pledge never to become complacent'

'I pledge I will develop the knowledge to do no harm with professional skills all wrapped up in a blanket of compassion'

'I pledge that I will never be influenced by bad habits'

'I will treat you as I would my loved ones'

'I pledge to put patient safety at the front of everything I do'

'When guarding someone's safety I will be the lion not the sheep'

Figure 10.1: Wall of confidence

Activity 10.6   *Reflection*

* With peers or colleagues, build your own wall of confidence, reflecting on your own beliefs and values about safety, harm-free care, risk and nursing.

As this activity is based on your own thoughts and ideas, there is no answer at the end of the chapter.

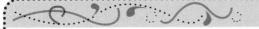

Chapter summary

This chapter has offered you an opportunity to reflect on your own skills and learning needs in relation to promoting patient safety and managing risk. It has also helped you to critically evaluate your own personal philosophies about nursing and patient safety. We have considered the recommendations made in light of recent safety issues and explored the potential way forward to improving patient safety. Together we may not be able to change the world overnight and right the wrongs in healthcare, but we can make a difference!

Activities: brief outline answers

Activity 10.2: Reflection (page 171)

Some nurses may not raise concerns because of the following: fear that they might be wrong, fear of putting their jobs at risk, intimidation by colleagues, bullying, reduced job opportunities, fear of being labelled as a 'troublemaker', not wanting to be a nuisance, or not wanting to be a moaner.

Activity 10.3: Critical thinking (page 173)

You could, of course, pass your concerns on to somebody more senior in the hope that he or she will approach Dr Bull. Some of you may feel confident to approach him yourself and point out that he has forgotten to wash his hands. Using well-developed communication skills will reduce the risk of you appearing confrontational. There is no guarantee you will receive a positive response from Dr Bull, but you are acting professionally and appropriately.

Activity 10.4: Reflection (page 174)

The following examples of risk assessment tools may have appeared in your answer:

- pain assessment;
- tissue viability assessment;
- nutritional assessment;
- moving and handling assessment;
- hospital anxiety rating scale;
- risk of self-harm.

Activity 10.5: Critical thinking (page 174)

You may have considered the following:

- good communication skills;
- assertiveness to ensure your concerns are heard;
- confidence in your own abilities;
- a good level of knowledge and evidence to underpin your practice;
- a sense of professionalism;
- ability to keep accurate records;
- well-developed interpersonal skills;
- good observational skills and an ability to 'notice';
- awareness of policy, legislation and procedure, local and national;
- ability to work autonomously and also with other team members;
- a clear sense of accountability and responsibility.

Further reading

Francis, R (2013) *Report of the Mid Staffordshire NHS Foundation Trust Public Inquiry. Executive summary*. Available at **www.midstaffspublicinquiry.com/report**.

This report summary is accessible and outlines the key findings and recommendations of the Mid Staffordshire Inquiry.

Lynch, J (2009) *Health Records in Court*. Milton Keynes: Radcliffe.

This provides practical legal advice in relation to record keeping, drawing on case studies to illustrate good practice.

Williamson, GR, Jenkinson, T, Proctor-Childs, T (2010) *Contexts of Contemporary Nursing*, 2nd edition. London: Sage/Learning Matters.

This book offers an insight into the varied factors that impact upon nursing practice. Nurses need to understand the political, educational and media influences in healthcare in order to deliver high-quality care.

Glossary

adverse incident   an untoward medical occurrence.

algorithm   a procedure or formula for solving problems.

autonomy   the power to govern oneself.

bundle see care bundle

care bundle   a tool that is used to help measure the application of good evidence. Care bundles are viewed as an approach to increase the reliability of delivering evidence-based practice.

checklist   a comprehensive list of important or relevant actions or steps to be taken in a specific order.

clinical governance   a systematic way of organising and maintaining quality in healthcare organisations.

error   a mistake.

five whys   a problem-solving analysis technique. A question-asking method is used to explore the cause-and-effect relationships underlying a particular problem. The primary goal is to find the root cause of a defect or problem.

hierarchy / hierarchical   categorisation of a group of people according to status or ability.

human error   an error caused by human factors.

human factors   how humans behave physically and psychologically in a number of situations.

Incident Decision Tree   a tree diagram or chart that can be used to determine a course of action in situations that could possibly have alternative outcomes. When two or more events have an effect on each other, different decisions, alternatives and possible outcomes are considered.

latent conditions   conditions that, when combined with other factors, allow active failures to occur.

litigation   a lawsuit.

London Protocol   a comprehensive and thoughtful process in relation to the investigation and analysis of critical incidents. Used by clinicians, risk and patient safety managers, researchers and others who want to reflect and learn from critical incidents, the protocol goes beyond the more usual identification of fault and blame.

medical iatrogenesis   health problem resulting from medical intervention.

near miss   action that just fell short of causing an untoward incident.

negligent / negligence   in the context of patient safety, relates to substandard practice.

never events   category of untoward incidents, mistakes and errors that should never occur.

paternalistic   refers to authority exercised to limit individual responsibility.

patient safety   keeping patients free from harm.

petechial   describes a small spot due to effusion of blood beneath the tissue.

sick day rules   guidelines for patients with diabetes providing advice on how to manage blood sugars and insulin / tablets during times of illness.

system failure   a number of failures in an organisation's system that lead to an incident.

untoward incident   a troublesome or adverse incident.

whistleblowing   raising concerns about a person or practices.

References

Advisory Committee on the Safety of Nuclear Installations (ACSNI) (1993) *Study Group on Human Factors, Third Report: Organising for safety.* London: HMSO.

Amalberti, R, Vincent, C, Auroy, Y and de Saint Maurice, G (2006) Violations and migrations in healthcare: a framework for understanding and management. *Quality and Safety in Healthcare,* 15(Suppl. 1): i66–7.

Association of Public Health Observatories (APHO) (2010) *Diabetes Prevalence Model for England.* NHS National Diabetes Support Team. York: Yorkshire and Humber Public Health Observatory. Available at www.yhpho.org.uk/resource/view.aspx?RID=81123 (accessed 9 March 2013).

Bach, S and Ellis, P (2011) *Leadership, Management and Team Working in Nursing.* Exeter: Learning Matters.

Baggot, R (2002) Regulatory politics, health professions and the public interest, in Allsop, J and Saks, M (eds) *Regulating the Health Professions.* London: Sage.

Baldwin, R and Cave, M (1999) *Understanding Regulation: Theory, strategy and practice.* Oxford: Oxford University Press.

Bergman, R (1981) Accountability: definition and dimensions. *International Nursing Review,* 28(2): 53–9.

Better Regulation Task Force (1999) *Self-regulation: Interim report.* London: Cabinet Office.

Bristol Royal Infirmary (BRI) (2001) *The Report of the Public Inquiry into Children's Heart Surgery at the Bristol Royal Infirmary 1984–1995* (Kennedy Report). Bristol: BRI.

Bromiley, M and Reid, J (2012) Clinical human factors: the need to speak up to improve patient safety. *Nursing Standard,* 26(35): 35–40.

Buykx, P, Kinsman, L, Cooper, S, McConnell-Henry, T, Cant, R, Endacott, R and Scholes, J (2011) FIRST²ACT: educating nurses to identify patient deterioration – a theory based model for best practice simulation education. *Nurse Education Today,* 31(7): 687–93.

Carr, S and Pearson, P (2006) Delegation: perception and practice in community nursing. *Primary Health Care Research and Development,* 6(1): 72–81.

Clarke, SP and Aiken, LH (2003) Failure to rescue. *American Journal of Nursing,* 103(1): 42–7.

Copping, C (2005) Preventing and reporting drug administration errors. *Nursing Times,* 101(33): 32–4.

Cuthbertson, BH (2003) Outreach critical care: cash for questions? *British Journal of Anaesthesia,* 90(1): 5-6.

Davies, C and Beach, A (2000) *Interpreting Professional Self-Regulation: A history of the United Kingdom Central Council for Nursing, Midwifery and Health Visiting.* London: Routledge.

Davis, RE, Koutantji, M and Vincent, CA (2008) How willing are patients to question healthcare staff on issues related to the quality and safety of their healthcare? An exploratory study. *Quality & Safety in Healthcare,* 17(2): 90-6.

Department of Health (DH) (1997) *The New NHS: Modern, dependable.* London: HMSO.

Department of Health (DH) (2000a) *An Organisation with a Memory.* London: The Stationery Office.

Department of Health (DH) (2000b) *No Secrets: Guidance on developing and implementing multi-agency policies and procedures to protect vulnerable adults.* London: The Stationery Office.

Department of Health (DH) (2007) *Saving Lives: Reducing infection, delivering clean and safe care*. London: Department of Health.

Department of Health (DH) (2010a) *Clinical Governance and Adult Safeguarding: An Integrated Process*. London: The Stationery Office.

Department of Health (DH) (2010b) *The NHS Outcomes Framework 2011/2012*. London: Department of Health.

Department of Health (DH) (2010c) *Equity and Excellence: Liberating the NHS*. London: Department of Health.

Department of Health (DH) (2012) *Liberating the NHS: Developing the healthcare workforce: from design to delivery*. London: Department of Health.

De Vries, EN, Ramrattan, MA, Smorenburg, SM, Gouma, DJ and Boermeester, MA (2008) The incident and nature of in-hospital adverse events: a systematic review. *Journal of Minimally Invasive Gynecology*, 16(4): 23–33.

Dimond, B (2011) *Legal Aspects of Nursing*. London: Pearson.

Donabedian, A (2003) *An Introduction to Quality Assurance in Healthcare*. New York: Oxford University Press.

Flin, R, O'Connor, P and Crichton, M (2008) *Safety at the Sharp End: A guide to non-technical skills*. Farnham: Ashgate.

Francis, R (2010) *The Mid Staffordshire NHS Foundation Trust Inquiry: Independent inquiry into care provided by Mid Staffordshire NHS Foundation Trust, January 2005–March 2009*. London: The Stationery Office.

Francis, R (2013) *The Mid Staffordshire NHS Foundation Trust Public Inquiry: Report of the Mid Staffordshire NHS Foundation Trust Public Inquiry: Final report*. London: The Stationery Office.

Gilien, P and Graffin, S (2010) Nursing delegation in the United Kingdom. *The Online Journal of Issues in Nursing*, 15(2). Available at www.nursingworld.org/mainmenucategories/anamarketplace/anaperiodicals/OJIN/TableofContents/Vol152010/No2May2010/Delegation-in-the-United-Kingdom.html (accessed 3 January 2013).

Glendon, AI and McKenna, EF (1995) *Human Safety and Risk Management*. London: Chapman and Hall.

Griffith, R and Tengnah, C (2010) *Law and Professional Issues in Nursing*, 2nd edition. Exeter: Learning Matters.

Haines, S and Coad, S (2001) Supporting ward staff in acute areas: expanding the service. *Intensive and Critical Care Nursing*, 17(2): 105–9.

Halm, M (2009) Hourly rounds: what does the evidence indicate? *American Association of Critical Care Nurses*, 18(6): 581–4.

Harmer, M (2005) *Anonymous version of the Independent Report on the Death of Elaine Bromiley*. Available at www.chfg.org/resources/07_qrt04/Anonymous_Report_Verdict_and_Corrected_Timeline_Oct_07.pdf (accessed 4 June 2013).

Healthcare Commission (2007) *Investigation Report: Maidstone and Tunbridge Wells NHS Trust*. London: NCC.

Health Foundation (2011) *Evidence Scan: Levels of harm*. London: The Health Foundation.

Hillman, K, Chen, J, Cretikos, M, Bellomo, R, Brown, D, Doig, G, Finfer, S and Flabouris, A (2005) Introduction of the medical emergency team (MET) system: a cluster-randomised controlled trial. *Lancet*, 366(9492): 2091–7.

Hughes, RG (2008) Nurses at the 'sharp end' of patient care, in Hughes, RG (ed.) *Patient Safety and Quality: An evidence based handbook for nurses*. Rockville, MD: Agency for Healthcare Research and Quality, US Department of Health and Human Services.

Illich, I (2002) *Limits to Medicine: Medical Nemesis: The expropriation of health*. London: Marion Boyars.

Institute for Innovation and Improvement (2008) *SBAR: Situation-Background-Assessment-Recommendation*. Available at www.institute.nhs/uk/quality_and_service_improvement_tools (accessed 9 June 2013).

James, D (2008) Inquest told of hospital death 'neglect'. *Western Telegraph*, 18 April. Available at www.westerntelegraph.co.uk/news/2207011.inquest_told_of_hospital_death_neglect (accessed 2 October 2013).

Jansen JO and Cuthbertson BH (2010) Detecting critical illness outside of the ICU: the role of track and trigger systems. *Current Opinion in Critical Care*, 16(3): 184–90.

Jones, S, Bottle, A and Griffiths, P (2011) An assessment of 'failure to rescue' derived from routine NHS data as a nursing sensitive patient safety indicator for surgical inpatient care. *International Journal of Nursing Studies*, 50(2): 292–300.

Lynch, J (2009) *Health Records in Court*. Milton Keynes: Radcliffe.

Mander, R (1995) Where does the buck stop? Accountability in midwifery, in Watson, R (ed.) *Accountability in Nursing Practice*. London: Chapman Hall.

McArthur-Rouse, F (2001) Critical care outreach services and early warning scoring systems: a review of the literature. *Journal of Advanced Nursing*, 36(5): 696–704.

McSherry, R and Pearce, P (2002) *Clinical Governance: A guide to implementation for healthcare professionals*. Oxford: Blackwell Science.

Meadows, S, Baker, K and Butler, J (2005) The Incident Decision Tree: Guidelines for action following patient safety incidents, in Henriksen, K, Battles, JB and Marks, ES (eds) *Advances in Patient Safety*, vol. 4. Rockville, MD: Agency for Healthcare Research and Quality.

Mencap (2012) *Death by Indifference: 74 deaths and counting. A progress report 5 years on*. London: Mencap.

Morgan, RJM and Wright, MM (2007) In defence of early warning scores. *British Journal of Anaesthesia*, 99(5): 747–8.

National Audit Office (NAO) (2004) *Improving Patient Care by Reducing the Risk of Hospital Acquired Infection: A progress report*. London: The Stationery Office.

National Institute for Health and Clinical (now Care) Excellence (NICE) (2007) *Acutely Ill Patients in Hospital: Recognition of and response to acute illness in adult in hospital*. London: NICE.

National Patient Safety Agency (NPSA) (2005) *Being Open When Patients are Being Harmed*. London: NPSA.

National Patient Safety Agency (NPSA) (2007a) *Recognising and Responding Appropriately to Early Signs of Deterioration in Hospitalised Patients*. London: NPSA.

National Patient Safety Agency (NPSA) (2007b) *Safety in Doses: Improving the use of medicines in the NHS*. London: NPSA.

National Patient Safety Agency (NPSA) (2007c) *Safety in Doses: Medication safety incidents in the NHS*. Fourth report from the Patient Safety Observatory. London: NPSA.

National Patient Safety Agency (NPSA) (2007d) *Safer Care for the Acutely Ill Patient: Learning from serious incidents*. Fifth report from the Patient Safety Observatory. London: NPSA. Available at www.nrls.npsa.nhs.uk/EasySiteWeb/getresource.axd?AssetID=60140&type=full&servicetype=Attachment (accessed 2 August 2013).

National Patient Safety Agency (NPSA) (2008a) *Resuscitation in Mental Health and Learning Disabilities Settings: A rapid response report*. London: NPSA.

National Patient Safety Agency (NPSA) (2008b) *Seven Steps to Patient Safety in Mental Health*. London: NPSA.

National Patient Safety Agency (NPSA) (2008c) *Significant Event Audit.* London: NPSA.

National Patient Safety Agency (NPSA) (2008d) *Foresight Training Resource Pack 5: Examples of James Reason's 'three bucket' model.* London: NPSA. Available at www.nrls.npsa.nhs.uk/resources/?EntryId45=59840 (accessed 20 July 2013).

National Patient Safety Agency (NPSA) (2011a) *What is a Patient Safety Incident?* Available at www.npsa.nhs. uk/nrls/reporting/what-is-a-patient-safety-incident (accessed 8 August 2013).

National Patient Safety Agency (NPSA) (2011b) *The Adult Patient's Passport to Safer Use of Insulin.* Patient Safety Alert. London: NPSA.

National Patient Safety Agency (NPSA) (2011c) NPSA releases Organisation Patient Safety Incident reporting data (England). Available at www.npsa.nhs.uk/corporate/news/npsa-releases-organisation-patient-safety-incident-reporting-data-england (accessed 10 October 2013).

NHS Diabetes (2010) *Safe and Effective Use of Insulin in Hospitalised Patients.* London: NHS.

Nightingale, F (1860/1969) *Notes on Nursing: What it is and what it is not.* New York: Dover.

Norris, B (2009) Human factors and safe patient care. *Journal of Nursing Management,* 17(2): 203–11.

Norris, B, Currie, L and Lecko, C (2012) The importance of applying human factors to nursing practice. *Nursing Standard,* 26(32): 36–40.

Northway, R and Jenkins, R (2013) *Safeguarding Adults in Nursing Practice.* London: Sage/Learning Matters.

Nursing and Midwifery Council (NMC) (2002) *Code of Professional Conduct.* London: NMC.

Nursing and Midwifery Council (NMC) (2006) *Accountability: A–Z advice.* London: NMC.

Nursing and Midwifery Council (NMC) (2007) *Standards for Medicines Management.* London: NMC.

Nursing and Midwifery Council (NMC) (2008) *The Code: Standards of conduct, performance and ethics for nurses and midwives.* London: NMC.

Nursing and Midwifery Council (NMC) (2009) *Record Keeping: Guidance for nurses and midwives.* London: NMC.

Nursing and Midwifery Council (NMC) (2010a) *Standards for Pre-registration Nursing Education.* London: NMC. Available at http://standards.nmc-uk.org/pages/welcome.aspx (accessed 7 June 2013).

Nursing and Midwifery Council (NMC) (2010b) *Raising and Escalating Concerns: Guidance for nurses and midwives.* London: NMC.

Nursing and Midwifery Council (NMC) (2010c) *Guidance on Professional Conduct for Nursing and Midwifery Students.* London: NMC.

Nursing and Midwifery Council (NMC) (2010d) *Standards for Medicines Management.* London: NMC.

Nursing and Midwifery Council (NMC) (2010e) *Safeguarding Adults: If you don't do something, who will?* London: NMC.

Nursing and Midwifery Council (NMC) (2011) *Advice and Information for Employers of Nurses and Midwives.* London: NMC.

Nursing and Midwifery Council (NMC) (2012a) *Nursing and Midwifery Council Annual Report 2011–12.* London: NMC.

Nursing and Midwifery Council (NMC) (2012b) *Midwives Rules and Standards.* London: NMC.

Nursing and Midwifery Council (NMC) (2012c) *Delegation: A–Z advice.* London: NMC.

Nursing and Midwifery Council (NMC) (2012d) *Raising and Escalating Concerns: Guidance for nurses and midwives.* London: NMC.

Oakley, J and Slade, V (2006) Physiological observation track and trigger. *Nursing Standard*, 20(27): 48–54.

O'Brien, M, Spires, A and Andrews, K (2011) *Introduction to Medicines Management in Nursing*. Exeter: Learning Matters.

Patient Safety First (2010a) *'How to' Guide for Implementing Human Factors in Healthcare*. London: NHS. Available at www.patientsafetyfirst.nhs.uk (accessed 4 March 2013).

Patient Safety First (2010b) *'How to' Guide for Reducing Harm from Insulin in Hospitals*. London: NHS. Available at www.patientsafetyfirst.nhs.uk (accessed 9 July 2013).

Qipp Safe Care Team (2012) *Delivering the NHS Safety Thermometer CQUIN 2012/13: A preliminary guide to delivering 'harm free' care*. London: Department of Health.

Reason, JT (1990) *Human Error*. New York: Cambridge University Press.

Reason, JT (1997) *Managing the Risks of Organizational Accidents*. Aldershot: Ashgate.

Reason, JT (2000) Human error: models and management. *British Medical Journal*, 320(7237): 768-70.

Reason, JT (2008) *The Human Contribution: Unsafe acts, accidents and heroic recoveries*. Farnham: Ashgate.

Richardson, B (2002) Investigating issues around vicarious liability. *Nursing and Residential Care*, 4(7): 348–50.

Robbins, SP and Coulter, M (2005) *Management*, 8th edition. Upper Saddle River, NJ: Prentice Hall.

Royal College of Nursing (RCN) (2006) *Supervision, Accountability and Delegation of Activities to Support Workers*. London: RCN.

Royal College of Nursing (RCN) (2010) *Principles of Nursing Practice*. Available at www.rcn.org.uk/development/practice/principles/the_principles (accessed 4 June 2013).

Royal College of Physicians (RCP) (2012) *National Early Warning Score (NEWS): Standardising the assessment of acute-illness severity in the NHS*. London: RCP.

Scriven, M (2000) *The Logic and Methodology of Checklists*. Available at www.wmich.edu/evalctr/archive_checklists/papers/logic&methodology_dec07.pdf (accessed 19 April, 2013).

Silber, JH, Williams, SV, Krakauer, H and Schwartz, JS (1992) Hospital and patient characteristics associated with death after surgery: a study of adverse occurrence and failure-to-rescue. *Medical Care*, 30: 615–29.

Taylor-Adams, S and Vincent, C (2004) *Systems Analysis of Clinical Incidents: The London Protocol*. London: Faculty of Medicine, Imperial College London.

Tsai, Y (2011) Relationship between organisational culture, leadership behaviour and job satisfaction. *BMC Health Services Research*, 11(98): 1–9.

Tyreman, C (2010) How to avoid drug errors. *Nursing Times*, 4 September. Available at www.nursingtimes.net/how-to-avoid-drug-errors/5018923.article (accessed 5 January 2013).

US Institute of Medicine (1999) *To Err is Human: Building a safer health system*. Washington, DC: National Academy Press.

Vincent, C (2010) *Patient Safety*, 2nd edition. Chichester: BMJ Books.

Wachter, RM (2012) Personal accountability in healthcare: searching for the right balance. *BMJ Quality and Safety*, 22(2): 176–80.

Wheeler, H (2012) *Law, Ethics and Professional Issues for Nursing: A reflective and portfolio-building approach*. Abingdon: Routledge.

Wong, CA and Cummings, GG (2007) The relationship between nursing leadership and patient outcomes: a systematic review. *Journal of Nursing Management*, 15(5): 508–21.

World Health Organization (WHO) (2004a) *World Alliance for Patient Safety*. Available at www.who.int/patient safety/worldalliance/en/ (accessed 9 April 2013).

World Health Organization (WHO) (2004b) *Patient Safety*. Geneva: WHO. Available at www.who.int/patient safety/about/en/index.html (accessed 1 July 2013).

World Health Organization (WHO) (2009) *Guidelines for Safer Surgery*. Geneva: WHO.

World Health Organization (WHO) (2010) Patient safety handout. Available at www.who.int/patient safety/education/curriculum/course5_handout.pdf (accessed 12 January 2013).

World Health Organization (WHO) (2011) *Patient Safety Curriculum Guide*, multi-professional edition. Geneva: WHO.

List of statutes

Deprivation of Liberty Safeguards

Domestic Violence Crimes and Victims Act 2004

Equality Act 2010

Health & Social Care Act 2008

Human Rights Act 1998

Mental Capacity Act 2005

Mental Health Act 1983

Mental Health Act 2007

Misuse of Drugs Act 1974

Public Interest Disclosure Act 1998

Social Care Bill 2011

Index